The
Carer's Bible

Amanda Waring

Souvenir Press

To Dee Chase, Elizabeth Purcell, and Julia Julia, all
who have cared for so many with such love.

To all those who care and will care and
to the carers of the future.

Contents

Foreword   v

Introduction   ix

1. How to Ensure Dignified Care   1

2. How to Support Personal Care and Daily Living   25

3. How to Care for Someone with Dementia   51

4. How to Care for Yourself and Prevent Burnout   86

5. How to Support Emotional and Spiritual Needs   103

6. How to Support Creativity and Activity   116

7. How to Care as Relatives for Loved Ones   140

8. How to Give Compassionate End of Life Care   178

Appendix: How to write a care plan   221

Afterword   225

Bibliography and further reading   229

Acknowledgements

My heartfelt thanks to all at Souvenir Press.

Deep gratitude
To the contributors whose expertise and personal testimonies
have enhanced *The Carer's Bible*: Cathe Gaskell, Caroline
J Benham, Mandi Randall-Cramp, Jo Whitehouse, Liz
Blacklock, Elizabeth Purcell and Ernest Hecht.

To all those wonderful carers, staff and elders that I have met
throughout my life, bless you for sharing some of your experiences for this book.

To all those who have supported me through my caring journey seen and unseen. To my family, friends, teachers, mentors
and extended family who have believed in me and encouraged
me through darker days.

and of course ... Thank you to my son Ben who cares for me ...

with love
Amanda Waring

Foreword

Amanda Waring has done so much to raise awareness of the need for dignity, compassion and kindness in care services, drawing on her personal experiences and a gift for communication. It is now five years since she published *The Heart of Care – Dignity in Action: a guide to person-centred compassionate elder care*. She is, without any doubt, well-qualified to build on her immense knowledge and learning to share understanding of the role of caring in this new book, *The Carer's Bible*.

Carers are vital partners in our system of social care. But sadly this is rarely acknowledged and, as a consequence, their contribution is not always valued as it should be. A recent report on 'The Human Rights of Carers in Northern Ireland' published in 2014 by the Northern Ireland Human Rights Commission stated:

> "Caring can be rewarding and fulfilling as well as demanding. What is important is the need for recognition of the role being played and the support that should be available and easy to access. Too often, obtaining support can simply be a further additional struggle to overcome.
>
> Carers are not a homogenous group. Carers can be all

ages from children to the very elderly who are looking after family members. Each carer is an individual who has his or her own story to tell and particular needs."

Whilst there is much that is shared about the experience of caring for a family member it is helpful to be reminded that every caring situation is different. People and their circumstances vary and every caring situation is a personal journey. It is my sense that *The Carer's Bible* is part of the personal journey of Amanda Waring. The reason the words are conveyed so powerfully is because we know that they are drawn from a wealth of personal experience – she really knows what she is talking about! She is able to use her knowledge of what it is like to provide personal care and support in ways to offer straight-forward practical guidance for others.

Amanda's story is well known: the experience of witnessing a lack of dignity and compassion in the care received by her mother and actress, Dame Dorothy Tutin, turned her into a reluctant, but strident, campaigner. As a campaigner she has turned a negative situation into a positive force to improve the quality of care of older people through her films, teaching and writing. She has used her own resources and networks, passion and charisma to make change. Her first film 'What Do You See?' which features Virginia McKenna makes use of the poem "Look Closer' by Phyllis McCormack and manages to convey in just 10 minutes so much about how important it is to always see the *person* in every caring interaction. To always see the person behind the presenting condition or frailty or confusion. I was proud to promote the film to innovative not-for-profit care providers within the membership of the National Care Forum and to encourage all Registered Home Managers to make use of the film in training their staff.

Keeping the individual at the heart of care is absolutely fundamental to best practice. In fact, best practice in social care is not possible without it.

Carers do make an immense contribution to society by providing care and support to family members and for some it is a lifelong commitment. We know that at least 6 million people in the UK are providing care and without them the system of social care would probably collapse. However, too often carers feel neglected and undervalued. Getting information at the right time and in the right way can be difficult for many carers. *The Carer's Bible* therefore makes an important contribution to the need for information. It is important to remember that most care takes place in private by people who may not actually define themselves as "carers". It is, for the most part, a personal thing and for many carers the term "care" probably doesn't adequately describe what they do, day in and day out. I believe that their contribution to personal well-being, quality of life and health is vital and deserves to be acknowledged as such.

Amanda's writing style makes it seem as though she is speaking directly to you. I have no doubt that *The Carer's Bible* will add significantly to our understanding about how best to offer emotional and spiritual support in practical ways. Her discussion of grief and loss is clearly informed by a depth of knowledge.

The book covers personal care and daily living, care planning, dementia and end of life care in a straight-forward way. The fact that chapters are devoted to emotional and spiritual needs as well as caring for yourself is an added bonus. I was especially pleased to see that Amanda has included a chapter on creativity and activity in the book. Given her own background in the creative arts she is uniquely qualified to highlight the contribution that art, in all its many forms, can make to personal well-being and quality of life. And this is true for both people receiving care and support as well as family carers.

Although the primary readership for the book is likely to be informal, or family, carers the contents will be just as relevant to paid professional carers. The fact that it is written from the perspective of a carer accentuates its value, in my view, as a source of continued learning.

The delivery of "compassionate dignified care" is a journey towards quality. A journey which has no end as our efforts to attain and maintain standards continue to develop. Our understanding of the importance of care and support to individual quality of life and well-being arguably is getting better all the time. This practical book is a valuable additional resource to the social care library. I hope it is widely read and its lessons used to make a positive difference to the lives of people in need of care and support.

Des Kelly OBE
June 2017

Introduction

Welcome!

My name is Amanda Waring and I am writing this book for you, the carer. Whether you are a professional carer or a relative caring for an elder loved one, I hope *The Carer's Bible* will be an invaluable and inspiring handbook to ensure that you give the best care that you can, whilst supporting yourself to do this. *The Carer's Bible* is easy to read and includes practical hints and tips, checklists, exercises, solutions to dilemmas, anecdotal advice, voices from the experts, and unique ways to deliver compassionate dignified care to older people right to the end of life, and after death. *The Carer's Bible* addresses spiritual and emotional needs and heartfelt ways to connect with those in your care.

If you are a professional carer my hope is that within these pages you find what you need to educate, motivate and reassure, whilst inspiring you to foster deeper relationships with those you care for. Please ensure that you read the section on **How to Care for Yourself and Prevent Burnout** for you are as important as the ones you care for. If you are a relative caring for an elder loved one please ensure you read the section on **How to Care as Relatives for Loved Ones** where I hope to walk you through your caring journey, addressing fears and anxieties, providing solace and support and to remind you that you are not alone.

How to use this book

I have grouped the material into eight sections that can be read in any order depending on your particular needs. Each section shares knowledge, ideas and best practices for your continued learning and understanding to best support those you care for and those you love.

HOW TO ENSURE DIGNIFIED CARE

Guidance and Tips on supporting the dignity of another, addressing thoughtless behaviour, understanding dignity breaches and dilemmas, protecting your dignity, whistle-blowing, upholding the dignity of those from the LGBT community and different cultures ...

HOW TO SUPPORT PERSONAL CARE AND DAILY LIVING

Guidance and Tips on intimate care, bedpans, bathing someone with dementia, dressing, teeth brushing, hoisting, mealtimes, appetite solutions ...

HOW TO CARE FOR SOMEONE WITH DEMENTIA

Guidance and Tips on positive communication and engagement, understanding their world, solutions to common issues and behaviours, supporting sensory challenges, support for night time issues ... Please note that in **each** section as well as in the section on how to care for someone with dementia there are hints and tips on dementia care.

HOW TO CARE FOR YOURSELF AND PREVENT BURNOUT

Guidance and Tips on ways to prevent burnout, recognising signs of compassion fatigue, re-igniting compassion, self-care daily check list, positive solutions to restore emotional and physical balance, how to keep motivated and sustain morale ...

HOW TO SUPPORT EMOTIONAL AND SPIRITUAL NEEDS

Guidance and Tips on recognising and addressing emotional needs at times of transition, providing spiritual and faith support, making things better, helping others feel needed, gratitude, heartfelt listening ...

HOW TO SUPPORT CREATIVITY AND ACTIVITY

Guidance and Tips for promoting well-being, creative arts, music as medicine, sharing meaningful activities for those with dementia, thinking outside the box ideas, keep on moving, learning new things ...

HOW TO CARE AS RELATIVES FOR LOVED ONES

Guidance and Tips on supporting a loved one with dementia and at end of life in their home or with you, taking positive steps, who cares for the carer, changing relationships, loneliness, when and how to get help. Understanding the stages of death and ways to ensure the "living" in the dying process, addressing regrets, end of life wishes, ways to provide solace and comfort, rituals and ceremonies to help grief and loss, transforming grief, helpful organisations, moving forward . . .

HOW TO GIVE COMPASSIONATE END OF LIFE CARE

Guidance and Tips on how to be with someone who is dying, pacifying fears, pain management, words to uplift, comfort and inspire, letting go, creating a peaceful environment, end of life care in dementia, forgiveness, physical care, the dying process, post mortem care, honouring and remembrance, supporting different cultures, thank you . . .

I have also provided an appendix on **How to Write a Care Plan**, which gives Guidance and Tips on practicalities and documentation, The Mental Capacity Act, what to do and what to avoid.

You may notice there is often cross-referencing and some gentle repetition. This is because the book is intended to be dipped into, rather than read straight through. I hope to ensure that important principles will not be missed and that the points arising from them will be understood and put into practice. Furthermore, I think it is important to indicate where the same point applies in a different context.

A personal reflection on my own journey with care and how I came to write this book

I was delighted to be asked to write *The Carer's Bible* after the success of my last book *The Heart of Care* for Souvenir Press. I realised that many of my roles and experiences in life have provided material and inspiration for me to draw on in the writing of this book. For this reason I have included in this book some personal material I first introduced in *The Heart of Care* where I feel it is particularly appropriate here and sometimes with extra details that throw a new light, as well as new material.

As a carer

I cared for both my parents till the end of their lives. I moved from London to West Sussex to be near them. I tried to give them the support that they needed but it was not always smooth sailing! My time with them was full of moments of love, frustration, laughter, despair, grief and healing. I learnt so much during that time, about them, myself, my limitations, my resilience, my fears and my capacity for love. My personal experiences help provide emotional, spiritual and practical support for you throughout this book.

As an elder care campaigner, filmmaker, author and trainer

After witnessing the lack of dignified care my mother, the actress Dame Dorothy Tutin, endured in hospital I sold my flat to make my short film *What do you see?* to train care staff about dignity and compassion in elder care. I was invited by the government to initiate the Dignity in Care campaign and since 2005 I have spoken and trained around the world on elder care and in the media on improving elder care. Throughout this book I am delighted to share quotes and frontline knowledge from the thousands I have trained. I have also been able to utilise the experience of dear colleagues that I have met throughout my campaigning and teaching to add to all sections. I hope you will feel inspired to place compassion and dignity at the heart of your caring and to read the important chapter on dignity often.

As a soul midwife and carer to the dying

I have sat with the dying since I was eight years old, when I used to be taken by my granny to sing at the bedside of those who were terminally ill in the hospitals where she volunteered. Even at such a young age I seemed to have an understanding of what was needed through sound and songs, or holding that person's hand. It was as if I had done this before. I was not frightened. As a teenager I continued to sing regularly to those in care homes and hospices to help bring comfort and ease to elders in their final days.

From my twenties onwards I have undertaken many trainings and initiations and spiritual rites of passage. I have worked with different traditions and faiths, which have enhanced my knowledge and understanding of working with the frail and dying. When working in my role as a death doula, or soul midwife, I feel it is an absolute privilege to do this work. In the caring for a loved one and end of life care sections I share some of the ways I use to help support a dying person and those who are left behind. I hope you will read often the section on **How to Support Emotional and Spiritual Needs** to enhance your end of life care too.

As a Celebrant

I have always wanted to change society's attitude to death and dying, to see if we could change the emphasis from the morbid aspects of death into a celebration of the transformational aspects of one's passing. From the time when I took my first funeral at the age of nineteen, becoming a celebrant provided me with that opportunity. As a celebrant I write and conduct funerals (and weddings and other rites of passages). In the caring for a loved one section I share celebration of life ceremonies, funeral wishes and grieving rites and rituals to support you as you support others.

I can see how, even from the trauma of my mother's undignified care, much positive good has come. I have found ways to improve elder care through my film, books, celebrant work or by just "being" with the dying. I can see the threads that have woven through my life bringing me to this point of writing *The Carer's Bible*. My wish is that *The Carer's Bible* be a practical source of comfort, connection and friendship to sustain you on your caring journey.

For info on my dignity, films and campaigning work please go to www.amandawaring.com. For info on my work as a Celebrant and Soul Midwife please see www.amandawaringevents.com.

AND LAST BUT NOT LEAST

Thank you
For all the care that you have given, and all the care that you will give.

On behalf of all those who may not be able to thank you due to dementia, ill health, incapacity, I want to give my heartfelt thanks for all that you have done, and all that you will do. To care for another human being is sacred and important work. They need you and this country needs you!

With gratitude
Amanda Waring

1

How to Ensure Dignified Care

As a carer, offering person-centred and dignified care requires you to be on a continuous and exciting journey of discovery, to keep learning, observing and listening, placing those you care for at the heart of all that you do. The rewards can be many. Research has shown that supporting the dignity of another brings valuable insights and greater satisfaction to the carer themselves. As carers we must value the intrinsic worth of others and preserve their dignity. Dignity is associated with that person's sense of respect, self-esteem, pride and self-worth. Dignified care places an emphasis on the benefit of mutually respectful care and the building of positive relationships. This can be done by learning to walk in the shoes of an older person and seeing their needs.

Please make dignity a conscious and integral part of all your interactions, by valuing the older person's active involvement in their own care, engaging with them, and asking what they may need.

Why is dignity important?

Research with the terminally ill has clearly shown that a personal sense of dignity can actually make the difference between a person's wish to live or die. In one study two thirds of dying people in a hospital setting felt that their dignity could be taken away from them by those who were caring for them. When a concern for supporting dignity is not present or dignity is thoughtlessly eroded the individual can feel demeaned, devalued, humiliated, less than, outraged, angered, depressed, worthless, useless, hopeless, alone, afraid, pitiful, lonely, isolated, withdrawn, even suicidal. There have been so many shocking stories in the media about elders enduring abuse and undignified care, and it is vital that you understand your important role in upholding and protecting the dignity of others.

Remember

There is an intimate connection between an older person's self-image and the way they are regarded by YOU. We have the ability to restore or destroy an older person's sense of their self-worth and dignity by our attitudes, so let us be aware if we may have fallen into the ageism trap.

CONSIDER

Perhaps you may be reluctant to use technology fearing an older person may shy away from it, or do you routinely attribute physical or mental symptoms like depression or aches and pains to the ageing process without looking for other causes. Are there any subtle behaviours that you have seen that may be considered ageist, how would you go about redressing this?

Ageism in society means that older people are continually discriminated against. Ageism amongst care workers can cause a disinterested, "care less", prejudiced and even abusive approach. That is why self-reflection is an important tool for you as a carer to reassess your practice and improve interactions.

Reflect on the following:

- What does being treated with dignity FEEL like to you?
- What does being disrespected FEEL like to you?
- When we look at things from a personal perspective it allows us to engage with elders in a compassionate and more meaningful way.
- Only focussing on medical needs ignores the spiritual richness of elderhood.

CONSIDER

The common belief is that dignity is treating others how you would wish to be treated. Reassess this from a more person-centred perspective, because dignity is treating others how THEY would wish to be treated. There may well be differences.

"I had to learn this early on because when I saw elders in my care upset I would automatically go to hug them, because that was what I would want if I was upset. I didn't stop to think to ask or consider that it might not be treating them with respect by invading their personal space. Now I always ask and respond in the way appropriate for them at that time, because sometimes they may want physical comfort and at others not, just like the rest of us."

Sammy, carer

Remember

You are not alone with dignity challenges you may face in your delivery of care. To provide a supportive forum for care staff and the sharing of good practice you can become a dignity champion. We on the dignity council are there to help you with issues as well as provide advice from fellow carers and professionals. Materials are available as useful reminders of how to give dignified care. Information and support can be found at www.dignityincare.org.uk.

Do

- have ZERO tolerance of all forms of abuse;
- support people with the same respect you would want for yourself or family;
- treat each person as an individual by offering a personalised service;
- enable people to maintain the maximum level of independence choice and control;
- listen and support people to express their needs and wants;
- respect people's rights to privacy;
- ensure people feel able to complain without fear of retribution;
- engage with family members and carers as care partners;
- assist people to maintain confidence and a positive self-esteem;
- act to alleviate people's loneliness and isolation.

To maintain dignified care means that you should continually assess, examine, and adjust your behaviour and communication methods.

Don't

- tell someone what they MUST wear, think how that might make someone feel robbed of choice, and control;
- leave someone in soiled undergarments or bedclothes;
- leave doors ajar when helping with personal care;
- tell someone what time they MUST go to bed, they are not a child;
- talk over someone or avoid eye contact;
- leave spectacles unclean, hearing aids without batteries;
- leave food or drink out of reach;
- leave someone wanting to go to the toilet;
- leave someone in pain;
- react to body odour or physical changes disrespectfully;
- speak down to an elder or assume an elder doesn't understand;
- coerce or bully an elder;
- give too many instructions all at once, or use medical jargon;
- give insufficient explanation;
- speak too fast;
- have illegible handwriting;
- use large childlike picture cards to help those with communication challenges to express their needs of going to the toilet, etc., please be aware that these can be on a key chain with smaller laminated pictures which can be more discreet and dignified;
- be too far away from the person or behind them when speaking to them;
- show a lack of interest in your tone of voice or body language.

CONSIDER

Consistent negation of someone's emotional state can alienate the elder and make them feel as if their emotions are "wrong". Telling someone not to be upset can become a subtle form of bullying that needs to be avoided so that an elder does not withdraw or become resentful or feel invisible. Good practice recognises, values and validates the emotions of that elder whilst all the while communicating "I am here if you need me. I see your pain, I will try and understand why you feel like this."

The world of a frail older person can shrink to perhaps ten feet around their bed, that is why you should recognise how the impact of your interaction and communication is amplified, a bed bound elder has no way to discharge or dilute the impact of any dismissive or disinterested interaction. There are real mental and physical health consequences to this behaviour and attitude including an impaired recovery from illness, increased stress and a shortened life span. So please don't raise your voice.

Tips for dignified communication

- Make sure you have introduced yourself. You may have a name badge but an elder may not be able to read it well or pronounce names that are foreign to them. It is very difficult for an elder to form a relationship with someone whose name they do not know and they may feel too shy to ask. Staff can unwittingly institutionalise themselves by becoming nameless and therefore faceless when they forget to introduce themselves regularly. Not only is it good manners but it will be reassuring to elders. For those with dementia, you may need to give prompts of your name more often whilst remaining patient and good natured.

- Check the elder has understood what you have said before moving on to the next topic.
- Ensure they have your focus and attention and eye contact.
- Use gestures and facial expressions to be more easily understood.
- Find a quiet area or room for private conversations and limit background noise.
- Do ensure you know how they wish to be addressed, what is their preferred name.

Remember

One of the best ways to improve your delivery of care is to ask the older person themselves. "Am I giving you the right level of support YOU need? How else could I improve my level of care?"

Dignity checklist

Recognise that good emotional care is as important as good medical practice. To lead with our heart and mind when ministering to others, to recognise the need for a balance of the physical and emotional needs, is to give good care. So, check in with yourself and your delivery of dignified care by answering the following questions, daily if needs be.

- How well have I adjusted my delivery of care to the ability of the older person. Have I made them feel rushed, confused or incapable?

- How well have I remembered to introduce myself? (See **Tips for dignified communication** above.)
- How well have I encouraged an older person to express their needs and wants?

  Consider

  Have you held back because you fear you won't be able to give them what they want, i.e. being in a residential home and the older person constantly wanting to go back to their own home? In the case of someone wanting to return home consider what you can do to make a feeling of "home" where that person is right now. Discuss ideas at a staff meeting.

- How well have I listened to their answers and have I been able to act on them, if not have I been able to find someone who can?
- How well do I respect a person's right to privacy?

  Consider

  Do I always remember to knock before entering an older person's room? Do I wait for an answer or at least wait for a short period of time before entering their private space? Even when they may be nearing end of life?

- How well do I engage with relative's concerns, how respectful am I of their opinions?
- How well do I manage my stress levels and still act in a polite and courteous manner?
- How well have I attended to personal care needs and how promptly?
- How well have I remembered to consider the habits, attitudes, tastes, moral standards, history, culture and spiritual beliefs of each person?
- How well have I recognised who that older person is inside, have I connected with them and involved them with their care?

  Consider

"Over Helping" can rob someone of their independence, no matter how well-meaning you are. Unless you ascertain what that person is able to do or wants to try for themselves they will shrivel to fit the box that you have put them in. Remember you are care partners working together with that individual.

BE AWARE

Apathy leads to neglectful behaviours and "benign incompetence" where carers can become blissfully unaware of what they are doing wrong. Dignity breaches exist in many care homes and NHS wards today. These include having the television on all day long, talking over or around patients, rushing mealtimes, leaving vulnerable adults exposed or soiled or with a lack of privacy, lack of stimuli in the room, being put to bed early for the ease of the team, lack of meaningful activity. All these work to create a sense of hopelessness and helplessness.

This demonstrates a culture of institutional and psychological abuse as staff are task orientated and routine driven; unwilling to think they simply do.

Recognising abuse

The older person's condition or history can put them at risk of abuse. These factors **don't** excuse abuse but they can put an older person more at risk:

- the intensity of their illness, disability or dementia;
- social isolation meaning the caregiver and elder are alone most of the time;
- the older person may have been an abusive parent or husband;

- the elder may have a tendency for aggressive behaviour physically or verbally.

*An older person can suffer **emotional** abuse including:*

- feeling intimidated through yelling or threats;
- being humiliated or ridiculed;
- being blamed often;
- being ignored;
- feeling isolated.

Changes in their personality or behaviour may be a sign of this

*An older person can suffer **sexual** abuse including:*
- being touched without permission;
- being shown pornographic material;
- being forced to undress.

Physical changes including bruises around genitals or breast, torn, stained or bloody undergarments, may be a sign of this.

*An older person can suffer **neglectful** abuse:*
- being denied the care that they need.

Changes in weight, bed sores, unsuitable clothing, dehydration may be a sign of this.

*An older person can suffer **financial** abuse:*
- having their case or belongings stolen;
- identity theft and forged signatures.

Unnecessary subscriptions, unpaid bills or missing items may be a sign of this.

IF YOU SUSPECT ABUSE REPORT IT. Make sure you know the procedures and protocols and organisations to contact as a professional carer or relative.

REPORTING CONCERNS

With thanks to contributor Cathe Gaskell, Director – The Results Company

A **whistleblower** is a person who raises a concern about a wrongdoing in their workplace or within the NHS or social care setting. "Whistle-blowers" have been involved in National Inquiries such as the Mid Staffordshire Inquiry, led by Sir Robert Francis QC, which led to widespread improvements in the health and welfare of patients across the UK and new laws to protect staff who raise concerns. In the NHS, each Trust has appointed a Freedom to Speak Up Guardian with whom you can raise concerns in confidence.

If you do not feel able to raise your concern with your immediate line manager or other management, consult your own organisation's whistleblowing policy, if there is one, and follow that. If you have tried all these, or you do not feel able to raise your concern internally, you can raise your concern in confidence with the Care Quality Commission who regulate and monitor care providers in the UK. The CQC takes concerns about patient safety very seriously and will act on concerns received. Concerns can be reported anonymously and the CQC will maintain your confidentiality.

You can call the Care Quality Commission on 0300 061 6161.

You can get free, independent and confidential advice from the Whistleblowing Helpline for NHS and Social Care on 08000 724725.

You can also call the independent whistleblowing charity Public Concern at Work for free and confidential advice on 020 7404 6609.

Complaints that count as whistleblowing

You're protected by law if you report any of the following:

- a criminal offence, eg fraud;
- someone's health and safety is in danger;
- risk or actual damage to the environment;
- a miscarriage of justice;
- the company is breaking the law, eg doesn't have the right insurance;
- you believe someone is covering up wrongdoing.

Do

- raise concerns locally as soon as you notice them, especially if they involve patient care;
- keep a diary detailing to whom you have told your concerns and what they promised to do to address them;
- maintain confidentiality if action is taken involving staff members that were involved;
- discuss concerns in your supervision or with a mentor, this is part of reflective practice and helps us develop our skills;
- remember you are protected by the law in reporting patient /resident concerns and there are people to support you when raising your concerns.

Don't

Ignore bad practices if you witness them. We have a duty of care to patients to act on our concerns and report them. If we witness bad practices that impact on poor patient care, this affects our credibility and potentially could cost you your job if later there is an investigation.

What if you're instructed to cover up a wrongdoing?

If you're instructed to cover up a wrongdoing, the person who tells you to do this is committing a disciplinary offence. If you're told not to raise or follow up any concern, even by a person in authority such as a manager, you shouldn't agree to stay silent. You should report the matter following the guidance of your workplace or professional body.

CONSIDER

You work as a care worker in a supported housing project for older people with learning disabilities. You become aware that even though your colleague is wearing gloves, she uses the same pair throughout her shift and doesn't wash her hands between tasks. For example, she prepares breakfast, delivers personal care, and writes in the hand-over book without taking the gloves off. This is putting the client's safety at risk and you have a professional duty to raise your concerns about this.

Tips for Carers

- Addressing concerns does not have to be undertaken by you, your role is to escalate concerns when you witness something that warrants them.

- Whistleblowing and safeguarding issues are often linked, make sure you are up to date in your safeguarding practices and can recognise abuse if it occurs and know where to report it.
- Attend updates on whistleblowing, raising concerns or the role of the Freedom to Speak up Guardian, so that you are up to date with the law and your responsibility in this area.

Further reading

www.cqc.org.uk

www.midstaffspublicinquiry.com/report

Understand your risk

It is difficult to take care of an older person who has many different needs just as it is difficult for that elder to struggle with infirmities and losing their independence. Both the demands of caregiving and the needs of the older person can create, in certain circumstances, situations where abuse may occur. The stress of elder care can lead to exhausted carers lashing out or neglecting those in their care. Carehome staff can be prone to elder abuse if they have a lack of training or too many responsibilities or are working in poor conditions.

Significant factors that may put us as carers at risk of elder abuse are:

- an inability to cope with stress and a lack of resilience;
- depression;
- lack of support;

- feeling our work as a carer brings no rewards;
- feeling helpless;
- feeling hopeless;
- feeling that we may be suffering abuse and a loss of dignity.

Please read the chapter on self-care and burnout. If you are at risk seek help from you GP, manager or carer's support group before things escalate.

Supporting dignity in different cultures

In our multi-cultural society it is important we all have tolerance and understanding of each other's backgrounds to ensure we maintain dignity and appreciate and learn from culture differences. Consider what you can find out about another's cultural background and share about yours.

Questions to think about can include the following.

- What are your/my customs and traditions?
- Who is in your/my family?
- What is your/my cultural perception of age and gender?
- What are your/my customs associated with food and dietary requirements?
- What languages do you/I speak?
- What festivals do you/I celebrate and what are their significant dates?
- How do you/I like to dress? Are there areas of potential offence?
- What are your/my religious practices, beliefs and values?
- What are your/my cultural attitudes to death and dying? Are there any special customs?

- What is your/my attitude towards intimate personal care?
- Is there anything else we would like to share?
- How long have you/I lived in the UK?

Adapted from National Activity Providers Association (NAPA) 2002 on providing activities for older people and used in *What do you see?* training pack by Amanda Waring and Rosemary Hurtley

Tips to celebrate difference

When I was making my documentary film *Can you see me?* I filmed a segment on end of life care and cultural diversity at St. Joseph's Hospice, who cater for a diverse community of many ethnic groups. They navigated their way through celebrating difference and working with challenges there by appointing leaders from the local ethnic communities to liaise often with the hospice. Prejudices and stereotyping were discussed and addressed and in the film I share their examples of good practice, which include these tips:

- bridge the gap – I hold a day of celebration of each culture and tradition, flags drawn, traditional clothing worn, food tasted, music played, dances tried, films watched, photos displayed, recipes shared, quotations from different religions and faiths;
- employ volunteer translators and use google translate apps to ease communication difficulties;
- ensure staff have learnt different meanings of specific gestures for different cultures, learning what may inadvertently cause offence in verbal and non-verbal communication;

- discover different greetings in different languages and use them appropriately.

Dignified care of the LGBT community

As carers we need to examine our own prejudices around sexual orientation. Spend some time in self-reflection on this subject, asking yourself: "Do I have a potential prejudice toward an elder who is lesbian, gay, bisexual, or transgender?" This awareness can assist you to work through any emotional responses, and prompt you to seek out appropriate information, help and support to ensure you are able to treat everyone with equality and dignity. It is important to be culturally sensitive to all elders, to be respectful of diversity, and give appropriate care.

Some lesbian, gay, bisexual and transgender people may be worried about receiving care services; for example, having to "come out" to home visitors or feeling judged by care workers. The Equality Act 2010 protects them from discrimination and this applies to care services too, which means they should always be treated with dignity when in care. Care should be offered by staff who will not judge them and with whom, over time, they feel able to talk openly.

In some cases, lesbian, gay, bisexual and transgender people may be put off asking for help and support because they are fearful of intolerant or insensitive reactions from strangers.

As social acceptance has grown, awareness of gender identity and sexual preferences has increased. Please ensure you get further training on this. The term "transgender" is used for individuals who don't identify with the gender they were assigned at birth.

*

"One concern in working with transgender patients is that the healthcare professional may offend the transgender patient. It is important to have open discussions with the person: "Which gender do you identify with? Do you prefer to be called a he or a she? What name do you prefer?" Some patients may refer to themselves by slang or derogatory terms. It is important for healthcare professionals to be aware of these self-references to decrease an unintentional reaction to the language."

**Australian Medical Student Association,
Global Health Conference 2014**

What LGBT people want from health and social care services

SAFETY: to have confidentiality respected, and a robust complaints procedure to deal with discriminatory behaviours and abuse. Institutional support and protection from homophobic, biphobic and transphobic abuse for older LGBT people who live in shared environments.

RESPECT: to be able to choose to be out and open about their lives without negative consequences affecting the services they receive and the way they are treated.

CULTURE: culturally appropriate services and support, which is linked into local LGBT communities.

AWARENESS: to be welcomed by services and professionals who are well informed about gender identity, sexual orientation issues and equality.

KNOWLEDGE: and understanding of their health needs, agencies addressing professional discriminatory judgements and assumptions. Increase awareness of the risks associated with diagnostic overshadowing and provide clear guidance and training for medical professionals.

Visit stonewall.org.uk, the LGBT equality charity. Acceptance without exception.

No time for dignity?

Time can be your friend and not always a barrier to giving dignified care.

- If every piece of paperwork, equipment, laundry, and all medicines, notes etc., were put back where they were supposed to be how much time do you think you could save?
  Consider
  Being respectful and mindful of putting things back where they should be, means you or any other staff you work with will have considerably more time to be with the older people.
- Be honest about timings with those you care for, otherwise they may lose their trust in you very quickly.
  Consider
  Once trust is gone it can be very hard to gain it back. So if you say you are going to be back in five minutes and you know you won't be, adjust your words to, "I will be back as soon as I can". If you continually break your promises you erode your own self esteem as well as the trust of an elder. It is especially important that you stick to times for medication to prevent any breakthrough pain for an elder and a feeling that you have forgotten them.
- When you are short staffed, call bells are going off left right and centre, how can you make the person you are

responding to for their call bell needs feel they are as important as everyone else?

Consider

Being centred, focused and calm with an elder helps them be calm and have greater clarity too. Use your time well, inform the older person that you may have only two minutes but for those two minutes "I am all yours, how can I help? It is better to be fully present with an elder for two concentrated purposeful minutes than to be with them for five distracted ones.

Your dignity protected

To promote dignity in care means that your dignity should be protected too. I encourage all care homes and elder care facilities to have a poster of some kind that says, "Our staff have the right to be treated with dignity at all times – most people respect this, thank you for being one of them". This is positively phrased but still a clear reminder to uphold the dignity of staff. Add the pictures of staff members to personalise this more.

My personal story of dignity

I witnessed the devastating effect that the lack of dignified care had on my Mother, the actress Dame Dorothy Tutin, whilst she was being treated for leukaemia in hospital at the age of 70. I saw the impact that the lack of compassion and respect from staff had on her mind, body and spirit. My strong, independent mother crumbled within days and she said she felt like a "caged animal". I moved my mother to another hospital because of this, and thankfully the staff were friendly, communicative and respectful and my mother's spirits rose helping her to face the challenges ahead. However all too often I saw elders treated as if they were second class citizens, rudely dismissed, and ignored in hospitals. This propelled me into a crusade to ensure that older people in care are treated with compassion and dignity.

I sold my flat to make my campaigning and dignity awareness film *What do you see?* in memory of my mother. I speak around the world and train carers with this award winning film. Its impact is powerful and profound. I believe that the personal story can say so much more than white papers or legislation can, for when people's emotions are engaged then change can happen much more quickly because they want it to. We all need a reminder to see the person inside, to look closer and see "Me".

So please consider seeing my short film *What do you see?* at www.amandawaring.com. It is based on the poem below written by a nurse Phyllis McCormack, who was dismayed at the behaviour of her colleagues on their geriatric ward. She originally wrote the poem anonymously in the hospital magazine for fear of reprisals. I have used that poem in my work with the dying since the age of nineteen and I am so grateful to her son Mike for giving me permission to make it into a film in 2005 and to use it in my books.

What do you see nurse,
What do you see?
What are you thinking
When you look at me?
A crabby old woman,
Not very wise,
Uncertain of habit
With far away eyes.

Who dribbles her food
And makes no reply;
When you say in a loud voice,
"I do wish you'd try."
Who seems not to notice
The things that you do,
And forever is losing
A stocking or shoe.

Who unresisting or not,
Lets you do as you will;
With bathing or feeding,
The long day to fill.
Is that what you're thinking,
Is that what you see?
Then open your eyes nurse,
You're not looking at me.

I'll tell you who I am,
As I sit here so still,
As I move at your bidding,
As I eat at your will.

I'm a small child of ten . . .
With a father and mother,
And brothers and sisters
Who love one another.

A girl of sixteen,
With wings on her feet;
Dreaming that soon,
A lover she'll meet.

A bride soon at twenty . . .
My heart gives a leap;
Remembering the vows
That I promised to keep.

At twenty-five now,
I have young of my own,
Who need me to build
A secure and happy home.

A woman of thirty,
My young now grow fast,
Bound together with ties
That forever should last.

At forty, my young ones
Have grown up and gone;
But my man is beside me
To see I don't mourn.

At fifty, once more . . .
Babies play 'round my knees;
Again we know children,
My loved ones and me.

Dark days are upon me,
My husband is dead . . .
I look at the future,
I shudder with dread;
For my young are all busy,
With young of their own,
And I think of the years
And the love I have known.

I am an old woman now,
Nature is cruel,
'Tis her jest to make old age
Look like a fool.

The body, it crumbles,
Grace and vigour depart,
There is now a stone
Where I once had a heart.

But inside this old carcass,
A young girl still dwells,
And now and again
My battered heart swells.

I remember the joys,
I remember the pain,
And I'm loving and living
Life over again.

I think of the years . . .
All too few, gone too fast,
And accept the stark fact
That nothing can last.

So open your eyes nurses,
Open and see . . .
Not a "Crabbit Old Woman",
Look closer . . . see "Me".
  ~ Phyllis McCormack ~

2

How to Support Personal Care
and Daily Living

"The doctor of the future will give no medication, but will
interest his patients in the care of the human frame, diet
and in the cause and prevention of disease."

Thomas Eddison

When I ask carers what they would find most difficult about
needing care themselves one day, there is a unanimous
response of a dread of personal care, needing help with the
toilet, bathing etc. None of them want to be exposed, vulnerable, or naked with another human being. How would
you feel if you needed this degree of care? Would you feel
embarrassed, or that your modesty was being compromised if
you had to be washed by strangers? Use your personal feelings
to motivate gentler, dignified and sensitive interactions during
intimate care.

Don't be afraid to ask the older person if there is anything you could do better in your approach, to help maintain their dignity and trust in you. Seeing things from their point of view will help you build a rapport. Their feedback will be valuable and help them feel part of the process instead of just a body to be "done unto".

Personal care

Your communication at this time needs to reflect an understanding of what the elder may be feeling during intimate assistance. They may fear the loss of privacy and independence. You can help to keep their dignity intact by allowing as much privacy as possible. For example, if someone is able to get to the toilet on their own, help them to do so and then leave the room, if possible, until you are called to help.

Do

- maintain a clean, hygienic environment when providing personal care;
- maintain an elder's confidentiality by keeping stoma bags hidden and out of sight in a locker for example;
- respond sensitively to odour, do not show a reaction to an elder that could humiliate them;
- check there is enough toilet paper;
- provide privacy, a screen can be used to add some privacy;
- respond promptly and sensitively to any necessary clean ups;
- ensure undergarments are clean and dry;
- wash your hands.

Don't

- leave an elder on a bed pan or commode for longer than necessary;
- leave bathroom doors ajar exposing an elder to others and compromising their dignity unless absolutely necessary due to space and your physical needs to assist adequately;
- use split back night dresses;
- use wrong sized underwear;
- leave elders wearing pads without underwear;
- use wrong sized pads;
- hoist elders without covers.

Personal care checklist

TIMELINESS

Elders who need assistance to use the toilet should be able to receive timely and prompt help, with appropriate safety equipment provided.

EQUIPMENT

Essential equipment to assist people to gain access to a toilet should be readily available, used in a way that respects the person's dignity and avoids unwanted exposure.

CLEANLINESS

All toilets, commodes and bed pans must be clean. An elder must be enabled to leave the toilet with a clean bottom and washed hands.

RESPECTFUL LANGUAGE

Discussions with elders must be respectful and courteous especially in regard to episodes of incontinence.

Taken from Behind Closed Doors campaign, British Geriatric Society Guidelines

Using bedpans

There are different kinds of bedpans and it may take a few attempts with different styles until the most comfortable one for that individual is identified. To get a person onto a bedpan, politely ask them to lie on their back with their knees bent so that you can place the bedpan under the buttocks. The older person can also roll to one side while you put the bedpan against the buttocks, and then have them gently roll onto their back.

Do

- Get the things you will need beforehand – gloves, clean and dry bedpan with cover, bed protector, laundry bag, toilet paper, towel and washcloth, disposal bags.
- Wash your hands and provide privacy.
- Put on gloves, then slide bed protector and bedpan under hips, and position the bedpan so it is firmly against the buttocks.
- Remove your gloves and wash your hands again when finished.
- Ensure that any damp skin is cleansed and properly dried after a person has used a bedpan. If not dried properly, damp skin can speed up the development of bedsores and pressure ulcers.

- Remember to clean the bedpan regularly with hot water and soap, and rinse the bedpan thoroughly each time you empty the contents.

Tips from carers

"I found putting baby powder at the top of the bedpan helped the person's skin from sticking to the bedpan."

Diane, carer

"I keep bedpans odour-free by rinsing with cold water and baking soda"

Mo, carer

Perineal care

Perineal care refers to the cleaning of external genitalia, surrounding skin, and buttock areas. Perineal care is generally performed during bathing, but for older adults who are incontinent or have a urinary catheter, you will have to do it more often to keep the skin healthy and free of infection.

Do

- Protect the older person's privacy when providing perineal care by covering as much of them as possible. This also helps to keep them warm.
- Wear gloves because your hands will be coming into contact with body fluids and this will protect you both.
- Raise or lower the bed to a comfortable working height.
- Position the older adult with their knees bent and legs slightly apart, unless there is some reason not to.
- Drape the area with a towel.

- Clean the perineal area from front to back
- Use a separate area of the washcloth for each area or a new washcloth if the one you are using becomes soiled.
- After you wash and thoroughly rinse each area, pat them dry to prevent skin irritation.
- If the older adult is continent, once you have completed perineal cleaning and drying, apply a barrier cream.

CONSIDER

Personal and intimate care can feel frightening and invasive to an older person. Do consider having a favourite song playing to relax them whilst you attend to personal care needs.

Remember

Ensure that you explain the needs for wearing any gloves, for example, "It's because I don't want to give you my germs". Without an explanation for your need to wear gloves an elder can feel as if they are untouchable, or so unclean you don't want to touch them. Remember how little human skin on skin touch an elder gets and how valuable caring touch and contact is.

Bathing

Bathing another human being is an extremely intimate and private practice of care. Thoughtful and kind interaction is required with clear focus on the person being bathed and respecting their wishes and levels of comfort. The ritual of bathing when managed well should be a relaxing and enjoyable experience. It is a place where worries can be washed away.

Tips

Do

- Consider having a low level screen in the bathroom that you can sit behind if you have to physically be in the room (because of risks of falls etc.) but allows an elder the opportunity for some privacy and normality.
- Consider feelings of modesty. Have extra flannels with which to cover an elder, larger towels and bubbles in the bath to protect modesty.
- Consider seeing if they wish to bathe in a bathing suit if they are able to wash intimate areas themselves.
- Ask the elder if they want to talk or would prefer peace and quiet or some music or listening to a recording of natural sounds.
- Ask permission before touching an elder.
- Find out how much they can wash themselves independently. If you take over aspects of personal care because you are rushed for time you can quickly rob someone of their dignity and autonomy.
- Use a favourite bath wash or a softer flannel, candles, bubble bath. If using oils be very aware of how slippery this can make things though.
- Test the water temperature with your elbows and ask the person if the depth and temperature of bath water is okay. Adjust water temperature often if required.
- Ensure towels are heated and soft.
- Prevent falls by ensuring you have wiped away any excess water off the floor around the bathtub or shower stall.
- Consider this intimate time, with permission, as an opportunity to gently move and exercise stiff and painful joints in warm water.

Bathing elders with dementia

"By stepping back and moving into the world of the person with dementia, we are less likely to disable them or make them feel afraid. The starting point is to understand how the dementia affects them, learn to communicate on a sensory and intuitive level and to move away from the *doing* to a more *being* approach. Caring is being able to connect with the person and help enable them to feel whole. We need to take our time to connect first, help them feel they have faith and confidence in us before we start. We cannot rush a person who has dementia, their ways of thinking and taking in information have slowed down and we need to bear that in mind. Only then can we consider to help them with their activities of daily living."

Jane Mullins, dementia nurse consultant

When it comes to bathing and showering, there is often a deeper reason, other than just "not wanting to", for someone with dementia's refusal to bathe. We need to sensitively understand their perspective. An older person who is not steady on their feet or has trouble stepping in and out of the bath tub may fear falling or slipping. Perhaps they have forgotten that they have not bathed or showered recently. The sound or feeling of falling water, steam and echoing bathrooms can provide too much of a sensory overload. They may feel exhausted or overwhelmed by the whole process and perhaps may feel the cold more acutely than others. An older person with dementia may not associate bathing with washing or getting clean and they may not understand or recognise the sensation of water. They may have arthritic pain or other pain that they can't express and that has not been adequately attended to. There can be great fear and concern that their privacy is being invaded and they are left vulnerable and unsure.

Try to understand these anxieties to ensure your approach is sensitive and empathetic, so that you can make bathing a more enjoyable, relaxing and therapeutic experience for someone with dementia.

Below are some tips to help you do this.

Tips

- Do not rush the experience, it should be relaxing where possible.
- Find out from the elder or family/advocates if they have any preferences, habits or anxiety around taking a bath. Taking into consideration a person's lifelong habits will help individualise the experience.
- Keep the room comfortably warm.
- Have all supplies ready before starting a bath.
- Let the elder hear the sound of the running water.
- Respect the person's privacy.
- Keep the older person covered whenever possible.
- Consider using tap limiters etc. to prevent burning. Check that the water temperature is comfortable.
- Soft relaxing music can be soothing.
- Use good communication. Identify yourself, ask permission and explain instructions carefully, using short sentences and emphasising key words, accompanied by a demonstration if necessary. Use body language and gesture with appropriate tone of voice to support what you are saying. Repeat as often as is needed.
- Always explain what will happen next, using simple respectful language.

- Use small talk and reminiscence to make the person feel included and involved.
- Provide the level of support appropriate to their capabilities; for example recognising objects and what they are used for can be a problem for elders with dementia. Start an activity such as using a flannel by demonstrating the washing movement yourself to prompt memory.
- Make sure there are plenty of warm towels to wrap them in afterwards.
- Wear latex gloves any time that you may come into contact with bodily fluids or faeces.
- Document what works well on the care plan.

Some points are from *What do you See?* training pack by Amanda Waring and Rosemary Hurtley

Tips from carers

"The resistance to shaving that many men display because they do not realise that they need to be shaved, disappears when shaving is accomplished the 'old fashioned' way with shaving cream and 'Old Spice' after shave lotion."

Namaste Care

My thanks to Joyce Simard, who founded Namaste in 2003 to be an organisation of care support, offering end of life programmes for people with advanced dementia. I have worked in hospices where Namaste programmes are used.

"A person who fights having a shower may follow you to the bathroom if you start singing and they may even join in."

Dave, carer

"Promising something nice afterwards like a favourite snack works for me."

Sophie, carer

Bed baths

Bathing someone in bed may be an appropriate option if the person you are caring for is unable to get in to a bath or shower. A bed bath is accomplished by filling a large bowl with water, prepared ahead of time.

Do

- test the water before using to make sure it is not too hot;
- have two basins of water, one filled with some mild liquid soap for washing and another with clean water for rinsing;
- have the flannels, soap and any cream you are using near the elder's bed, along with a comb and brush;
- wash one body part at a time with a sponge or washcloth, and keep the rest of the body covered with a warmed bed sheet or large, warm towel;
- keep the elder's change of clothing close by;
- make sure to keep the room at a comfortable temperature.

Using a hoist

Make sure you have had the specific hands on training you need before using a hoist with an elder. Meeting the mobility needs of people is one of the most important things we can do, making the person feel comfortable, minimising discomfort and pain, while trying to encourage the person to be independent and keep a feeling of self-worth. Communicating and being empathetic to the person's individual needs, wishes and preferences can make their experience so much better. BUT we must be aware of the level and type of communication that the person can understand.

When using the hoist, a sling and other mobility equipment, we must consider personalities, conditions and past experiences of the person being moved.

Do

- Look at their face for communication of discomfort;
- ensure the sling is the correct size and fitted correctly;
- always have a minimum of two staff for good practice;
- look at the individual's needs;
- sing a song, gesticulate, as actions speak louder than words;
- communicate well, they may be very frightened;
- use a closed hand for the person's comfort.

Don't

- suspend a person in a sling while delivering personal care;
- use a toilet style sling on a person without core stability;
- use a standing hoist with a person with dementia, or someone who is unable to hold on with both hands/ weight bear with both legs (i.e. someone who has had a stroke);
- talk over them while moving the person;
- transfer anyone any further than a distance of six feet.

"On rolling side to side to place the sling underneath a lady with early stage dementia, she would shout, swear, scream and dig her nails into the carers that were trying to help her. She was up high on the profiling bed, as she looked down to the floor which must have felt a very long way away, she said 'don't let me fall down them stairs again'. The brain does funny things sometimes to protect us from harm, it hangs on to a memory which may come flooding back at any time to make us fear or stop us from falling or coming to harm."

With thanks to Mandi Randall-Cramp, Trainer, Sonnet Care Homes

Teeth brushing

Remember that you can feel very vulnerable when someone asks you to open your mouth. If I ask you to open your mouth now and keep it open for twenty seconds, are you comfortable? Do you feel exposed? Now imagine you had to do this in close proximity to a stranger, would you feel anxious, worry that your breath smells, be unsure? An elder can feel all of this and more. An older person may resist help with teeth brushing because perhaps they gagged when someone tried to do it before. Perhaps a previous carer, in their rush, forgot to wet the toothbrush and applied toothpaste to dry bristles hurting sensitive gums.

Try and ascertain what anxieties there may be and ways to reassure and alleviate them. If they have dementia and their taste-buds have changed, they may dislike the taste of the tooth paste so seek out other flavours like fennel or calendula.

They will need you to walk through every step with them with patience and clarity.

Tips

- Think about how and where it may be easier to brush their teeth.
- Brushing teeth does not need to be done standing at a bathroom sink, it can be done just as easily at a table with a towel, bowl and cup of water.
- Keep it simple and comfortable. Tell, show, do, to allow people to understand the process.
- Remember traditional toothpaste may have an unfavourable taste for some elders and may bother those individuals with swallowing problems, so try fennel or calendula.
- Use a toothbrush that has soft bristles and is easy to hold. *Consider*
  A child's size toothbrush, a powered toothbrush (which has a large handle and may be easier to use), or making changes to a toothbrush (depending on the ability to grasp the toothbrush handle) such as wrapping the toothbrush handle in a small face cloth.
- Replace the toothbrush as soon as it appears worn.
- If the person is in a wheelchair, it may be easier to stand behind them when helping with tooth brushing.
- If sitting knee to knee is comfortable then it will be easier for you to see into the elder's mouth when not brushing teeth at a sink or in front of a mirror.
- Remember to brush very gently along the gum line.
- Always check along the folds between the teeth and the cheeks where food can remain and consider gently swiping this area with a gloved finger or swab.
- For a person with part dentures remove them before brushing the teeth.

Denture care

Badly fitting dentures can lead to health concerns for older people, causing them to modify their diets to help make chewing easier and less painful. They may avoid healthy foods that have a tough, coarse or crunchy texture in favour of easy to masticate desserts and soups. They may stop eating the highly nutritional food their body requires, leading to malnutrition.

Do

- Check dentures regularly for cracks.
- Be aware that dentures shouldn't click when the elder speaks or eats. If they do they may need repair.
- Check the elder's mouth and gums for any signs of irritation or mouth sores as a result of ill-fitting and rubbing denture plates. Ill-fitting dentures can cause gums to bleed or become painful and sores can form. When they become painful, elders may stop eating or stop using their dentures.
- Remember dentures should be cleaned every day, brushed with a soft bristled brush to remove debris and food plaque.
- Brush gums, tongue and palate before the dentures are worn to keep them clean and free from potential irritants.
- Use a minimum amount of denture adhesive if needed, removing adhesive daily as you clean.
- Clean dentures over a towel to prevent breakage if they drop in the sink or on the floor.
- Store dentures in a denture container with water to keep them moist and prevent them from getting too dry, or losing their shape.

Don't

- Use normal toothpaste or bleach as both are too abrasive and may cause discolouration, instead use commercial dental cleansers or if not available mild washing up liquid. Ultra-sonic cleaners can be helpful too.
- Use hot water for dentures as that could cause them to warp.

Taken from the National Institute of Dental and Craniofacial Research (www.nidcr.nic.gov) and Tooth brushing Tips from the Muscular Dystrophy Association (www.alsn.mda.org).

Looking good feeling good

Do not forget to ask an elder if they would like help with putting on make-up, or brushing their hair, or doing their nails. Ask the men what grooming they may like. Men may need a shave, a woman may want her legs and underarms shaved. Be sensitive in your approach and allow for people's needs and likes to change daily. You may assume that if a person is dying or unwell they may not want to be bothered with such things, but conversely this might be the time when they would like help to make themselves feel better by looking better. In fact they may refuse to see visitors because they do not feel their appearance is up to their usual standard, so help them keep connected to others by tending to their desire to look good.

Helping someone with dementia to get dressed

Remember occupational therapists offer helpful advice for extra daily living support. When someone has dementia, try not to overwhelm them with too much clutter and choice which may only serve to confuse them further. Perhaps velcro could be used to replace buttons, and clothes laid out in the order they are to be put on. Use of labels, pictures and whole outfits together provides simple choices.

Assisting with mealtimes

Carers and elders sharing mealtimes together can be an enriching and social time. However assisting someone to eat a meal requires discretion and sensitivity to ensure you do not rob an elder of their sense of self belief or dignity. Appetite and the experience of mealtimes change as people age or progress through various stages of illness. As a carer it is important that you are able to recognise and support the fluctuating changes, all the while remembering that mealtimes should be an enjoyable event.

You could ask the older person what they particularly enjoy about mealtimes or share favourite recipes together. You could try to find out what special memories they have that are associated with food, for example Christmas, religious holidays, birthdays, or growing their own vegetables. They might enjoy having themed meals from different countries. The music and culture of the region could provide inspiration for conversation topics. Be creative and energised around mealtimes and try and involve the older person in the preparation of a meal in however small a way to help them feel valued and able to contribute by helping you.

Staff and residents eating together contributes to a family atmosphere in care homes, which provides a great opportunity for people to get to know each other in a relaxed way.

Tips for increasing appetites

- To help with a diminished appetite consider serving portions on a much larger plate to help the portion size appear smaller.
- Serving tiny canapés or tasty morsels an hour before a meal has been shown to increase appetite too.
- Making food appetising is especially important for those who find eating a challenge, have problems chewing or tasting or who may be feeling unwell or depressed. They need nutritious and attractive meals with the right sized portions presented on the plate.
- If an older person can only eat pureed food consider using moulds so that instead of an unattractive and undignified mush, the pureed food can resemble the food it actually is.

"I found it hard to decipher what was the real cooked English breakfast or its pureed counterpart the moulds were so good and the residents now love the new presentation and are eating more with greater enthusiasm."

Maureen, carer

Check list to make mealtimes a more dignified experience

Discover what you can offer to help them eat independently or more comfortably.

- Use equipment – consider what might be needed to assist someone with painful joints or arthritis. To prolong independence ensure you have specialist equipment, non-slip mats, large handled cutlery, to help grip. A plate

with a lip/guard for an elder who only has the use of one
hand.

- Observe – assess their needs and then ask an older person
  if they need any assistance so as not to rob them of dignity or their sense of control.
- Encourage – gentle persuasion must not give way to
  bullying.
- Enable choice – but ensure you do not give more than
  two choices at a time unless you have visual reminders,
  for frailer older people are likely to only remember the
  first or last thing you have said.
- Foster independency – for example offer an older person
  jam to spread on toast themselves, or sugar to stir into
  their coffee if they are able to do so. Do not take over.
- Consider presentation – if pureed food is required consider
  the creative use of moulds to make the food more appetising. Serve food on a larger plate to encourage an elder to eat
  more and not be overwhelmed by perceived portion size.
- Ensure no childlike bibs are used – clothes protectors or
  large napkins are more dignified.
- Give complete attention – silence mobile phones and
  other distractions. Be engaged and interested.
- Validate feelings – feelings matter so much. Empathetic
  listening and conversation are to be encouraged.
- Prompt where needed – if an elder has a memory problem remember to prompt at each step, only providing
  help if necessary.
- Allow enough time – feeling rushed not only erodes
  self-confidence but can force an elder to become more
  dependent, or give up trying altogether. DO NOT LOAD
  ANOTHER SPOONFUL BEFORE AN ELDER HAS
  FINISHED THE PREVIOUS ONE. Remember the
  right pace of care promotes independence.

- Tidy up – ensure an elder has finished and any messes or spills are gently, sensitively and discreetly dealt with.
- Consider seating – ensure your chair is not higher than an older person, which can seem intimidating to the frail elderly especially if you are assisting them, and never stand over an elder when helping.

Some points are from *What do you See?* training pack by Amanda Waring and Rosemary Hurtley

Remember

Don't

- leave food or drink out of the reach of an older person, a common mistake in hospital and care settings;
- clear away food without ascertaining if they were physically able to eat their meal or needed more assistance from you.

Dementia care and eating difficulties

An older person with dementia will have additional difficulties at mealtimes, so let's examine some challenges and solutions Challenges may include the following.

- Not being able to express their wishes – use visual aids and menus with pictures, ascertain from family members any particular eating habits or food preferences.
- Not recognising food or eating utensils and forgetting how to use them – try eating with the person with dementia, encouraging interaction, and you may even

find they copy what you eat and drink and what utensil you use, keep patient.

- Not having good motor skills – check that any glasses aren't too heavy or troublesome to grasp, use double handed beakers if necessary, lighter glasses and/or coloured drinking glasses, non-spill cups and easy grip cutlery. Ensure they are sitting upright and help them guide the food to the mouth if needed, always being mindful of and assessing varying daily levels of capability and the need for independence.

- Not having clear vision – ensure the room is well lit to enable them to see better. Patterned plates are confusing for those with dementia, consider using different coloured food and contrasting coloured plates and cutlery to enable clearer identification. Explain and describe what food they have on their plate so they can envision it before tasting it. Keep their drink in their line of sight and describe the drink to them.

- Not coping with background noise – let them decide where they would like to eat and limit background noise, including dishwashers etc., wherever possible, so that the environment is calm.

- Not having a good appetite – consider changing medication that may affect appetite, check for pain and discomfort, which may suppress their desire to eat. Consider sore gums and check dentures. They may be constipated or suffering from depression. Use finger foods or small snacks on a regular basis. Check that food is not too hot or cold, which will affect appetite. Serve one course at a time, small portions on a larger plate will seem less overwhelming. Music and nature sounds can sometimes promote appetite, elders may enjoy food linked to childhood memories or a particular time in their life. Keep food healthy and well balanced to protect their physical and mental well-being. Use spices and aromatics to enhance flavour.

- Not having good swallowing reflexes – soft and moist food works better, scrambled eggs, mashed potato, soups, jellies, ice cream. Gently stroking the larynx in an upward motion may prompt a swallowing reflex.

Peg feeding

Be aware when peg feeding – if this is not being done over-night – to remember this is the way that the individual has their meal. If no consideration is put into making the start of the peg feeding a special experience people can easily feel de-humanised. Find out if the elder wishes to start their peg feeding with everyone else in the dining area. Have you offered the latest mouth wipes that can be different flavours and be pleasurable for some? Can flowers be laid out or music played when a peg feed is started in an elder's room? Ask the individual what they would like.

Taken from "Doing it Well", guidance from the Beth Johnson Foundation written by Amanda Waring

Remember

The power of wholesome food to heal and restore both the body and mind cannot be underestimated. Wherever possible ensure that elders are nourished with good food to enable them to benefit from the vitamins and minerals that nature provides.

"Let food be thy medicine and medicine be thy food."

Hippocrates, born 460 B.C.

Assisting elders as a home care worker

As a home carer, or domiciliary carer, caring for an elder in their own home, your aims should be to develop and promote the independence of the individual by encouraging them to do as much for themselves as possible, helping them to live independently and have as much control over their lives as possible. You may carry out different tasks for each unique individual and provide support in a way that meets their specific needs, undertaking personal care, or household tasks e.g. laundry, preparing meals, cleaning. Other tasks may include shopping, collecting prescriptions and taking the elder to appointments or social activities. You will help to maintain a healthy and safe environment for that elder. Your very important role enables them to have the best quality of life and to participate in society as an equal.

Do

- Follow the fundamental standards of person centred care, dignity and respect and the need for consent.
- Remember that you are in their home and treat it with the respect it deserves.
- Ask your client how they wish to be addressed and put this into action.
- Ensure that those receiving your care are at the centre of all decisions and everything must be done in THEIR best interests, above that of their family or next of kin.
- Understand why professional boundaries are important.
- Remember that you are the elder's advocate.
- Provide the elder with dignity and respect in all aspects of their care.
- Ask the elder's permission before carrying out tasks that affect them.

- Follow correct working procedures as agreed by your workplace and the elder's care plan.
- Be aware of dietary needs, working with the care plan, ensuring elders have the right equipment and conditions to eat.
- Remember when there is no direct supervision it is very important that you as a lone worker are safe and that your self-assessment is accurate and your recording on care plans exemplary.

"Do talk to your client, sing with them, laugh with them and maybe even cry with them if appropriate. Talk about yourself, your family, hopes, aspirations. You may be the only contact with the 'outside world' or touch of normality that your client gets in the day. Do remember and be aware of when you need extra support – this is a sign of strength not weakness and in the long run this will stand you, your clients and company in good stead."

Liz Blacklock, CEO, Lapis Domiciliary Care

Don't

- forget to introduce yourself and smile;
- make assumptions about the elder, your way may not be their way;
- forget that if you have been delayed and you are going to be late you should let the elder know, or ask somebody else to do this for you;
- forget to make sure someone knows where you are at all times when on duty;
- do anything you are not confident in or trained appropriately for; you will put both yourself and your client at risk;
- be afraid to say no.

With thanks to contributor Liz Blacklock, CEO, Lapis Domiciliary Care

Reminders

FIRST AID KITS

First aid regulations 1981 state that the employer must make adequate first aid provision for all employees. In the workplace this means providing sufficient first aid kits, first aiders and a means of reporting and recording accidents or incidents. For you as a lone worker this means providing a first aid kit, this may be a one person travel kit to keep in your car or bag. Ensure you have this.

FORMS AND EMERGENCY NUMBERS

You will need forms for recording accidents/incidents and emergency phone numbers.

EQUIPMENT CHECKS

When you work in an older person's home you will need to ensure you carry out regular checks on any equipment you may use and report any faults or concerns. Your employer should risk assess any equipment you will be expected to use and provide training if needed.

PERSONAL PROTECTIVE EQUIPMENT

Your employer should provide you with gloves and aprons where needed but it is your responsibility to wear them when required. If you choose not to use them and your health or safety suffers this will remain your responsibility.

HAZARDOUS SUBSTANCES

The ones you will come into contact with are most likely to be cleaning fluids, medications, bodily fluids, hot liquids. It is your responsibility to wear appropriate personal protective equipment and make your employer aware if you have any allergies.

Report incidents or any type of injury, dangerous occurrence or death to your line manager so that they can ensure it is recorded and reported as required. For a full list of reportable incidents and details of how and when to report go to www.se.gov.uk/riddor.

3

How to Care for Someone
with Dementia

"Being unwanted, unloved, uncared for, forgotten by
everybody, I think that is a much greater hunger, a much
greater poverty than the person who has nothing to eat."

Mother Theresa

During the journey of caring for someone with dementia,
there will be joy, spontaneity, laughter, love, but there will
be darker and challenging times too. This section is to help
you navigate your way through, and actively support those
with dementia who may be struggling with the changes that
lie ahead. The positive strategies and hints and tips will guide
you through some of the issues you may face.

To care for someone with dementia we need to learn to
enter their reality and know as much as possible about that
person, their background and the things that matter most to

them. As well as having an understanding of what people with dementia might need, it is also important to ensure that they have us as carers to walk alongside them as they try to express themselves, knowing that we accept them for who they are at that moment. Someone with dementia will see the world differently to us and may move through different timezones and worlds which can be daunting for a carer, however it can also be liberating, and at times exciting too.

It can be easy to make wrong judgements or even try to "fix" their confusion rather than relieve their tensions and fears, so we must have an understanding of the psychological as well as the physical aspects of dementia. Our lives can be enriched through caring for those with dementia, so be open to the experience of learning with your fellow dementia time travelers: it may be a bumpy but exhilarating and insightful ride.

Living with dementia does not mean an end to living with hope, dignity and self-empowerment. Members of The Gathering Place in Seattle, a group of elders who are living with early-stage memory loss, wrote the following empowering message of hope to inspire other elders with early-stage dementia: "We have learned to live with our memory loss and still have productive lives with family and friends. We would like to give you hope that you too can live a full life. There will be obstacles to come, but you have an opportunity to give back to your community and yourself, and to experience beauty, happiness, and kindness."

PLEASE NOTE

Dementia care tips and advice are in every section of *The Carers Bible* for you to read.

Understanding dementia

There are five main types of dementia, but every type has one thing in common, a loss of intellectual abilities, which is not a normal part of ageing and becomes progressively worse as time goes on.

ALZHEIMER'S DISEASE

Alzheimer's disease is the most common cause of dementia or loss of intellectual function, among people aged 65 and older. The disease takes its name from a German neurologist, Alois Alzheimer. It is a progressive, degenerative disorder that attacks the brain's nerve cells, or neurons, resulting in loss of memory, thinking and language skills, and behavioural changes.

LEWY BODY DEMENTIA (LBD)

This is one of the most common types of dementia, after Alzheimer's disease. It usually happens to people who are 50 or over. There are two types:

- **Dementia with Lewy bodies** often starts when you have a hard time moving your body. Within a year, memory problems that are similar to Alzheimer's disease occur along with changes in behaviour and possible hallucinations;
- **Parkinson's disease dementia** first causes movement problems. Trouble with memory happens much later in the disease.

VASCULAR DEMENTIA

Vascular dementia affects different people in different ways, typically the symptoms can begin suddenly for example after a stroke. Symptoms are similar to other types of dementia such as Alzheimer's but they may particularly experience physical weakness, seizures, incontinence, psychological symptoms, becoming more obsessive, acute confusion, depression.

HUNTINGTON'S DISEASE

The earliest symptoms are often subtle problems with mood or mental abilities. It is an inherited disorder, as the disease advances uncoordinated, jerky body movements become more apparent. Physical abilities gradually worsen until coordinated movement becomes difficult and the person is unable to talk.

PICK'S DISEASE

Pick's Disease is one of the rarer types of dementia. The changes in personality allow doctors to distinguish between Pick's disease and Alzheimer's disease. There may be behavioural changes such as:

- intense restlessness;
- impulsiveness, poor judgement;
- overeating, craving unfamiliar foods;
- being rude when formerly polite;
- inattention to personal hygiene;
- loss of sexual inhibition;
- aloofness from others; loss of interest in things around them;
- rapid mood changes.

Websites consulted: Web MD, Wikipedia, Clinical Partners

"Carers may not always know what type of dementia the person has and if they did know, it will be a different experience for different personalities. We watch, we observe, we learn, we look at life history as it makes and shapes us, we look at different approaches, what helps, what upsets the person and we share that within our team. Behaviour charts should be used positively, not just when someone has displayed a negative behaviour, but a positive happy reaction, so we learn and progress positively in the person's world, their bubble."

**Mandi Randall-Cramp,
Sonnet Care Homes**

Typical aspects of behaviour in dementia

All behaviour is meaningful and needs to be understood, not simply "managed". People with dementia come to rely less on thinking and more on feeling, so providing emotional care is vital, and that means giving of yourself emotionally to support those in your care.

Typical behavioural aspects in those with dementia may include:

- confusion and disorientation;
- forgetting names and places;
- repeating oneself;
- wandering;
- being unable to hold a discussion;
- being unable to independently mobilise;
- hitting out and aggression;
- walking around all the time;

- uninhibited behaviour;
- not cooperating when being helped;
- constantly repeating the same thing;
- shouting or screaming.

"It's the unknown that scares me"
Charles (diagnosed with Vascular dementia)

"I can't do right for doing wrong"
Ginny(diagnosed with Pick's disease)

"It's the forgetting me I am worried about"
Norman (diagnosed with Alzheimers)

"It's really strange when you don't know what's real and what isn't"
Sandra (diagnosed with Lewy body dementia)

Understanding the losses

Understanding helps us not to judge but to validate feelings and assist where we can. How can we reach people from their world, rather than ours? What can we do to alleviate their pain and anxiety?

Best-selling author Terry Pratchett, who delighted so many with his fantasy creation the Discworld, had a long battle with early-onset Alzheimer's. He was very open about his experience and contributed a great deal to public knowledge, even making a film for the BBC. He tried to remain cheerful but at times it was clear how difficult it was for him to feel that he was slipping away little by little and could only watch it happening.

An elder needs your support and understanding to help them cope with the many losses they may have to endure:

- the loss of intellectual capacity including short term memory loss and the ability to make logical connections;
- the loss of communication skills due to poor concentration and language difficulties;
- the loss of certain senses;
- the loss of independence – problems with getting lost, needing supervision for activities;
- the loss of self.

These losses combine to create frustration, depression, anxiety, low self-esteem and fear for the future. You can support their self-belief by offering that person plenty of praise and encouragement, celebrate successes and focus on the positives. To provide the best quality care that you can for that person means recognising that it is not an unchangeable illness where nothing further can be done, but with your support their well-being **can** and **will be** improved.

"I have dementia but it doesn't have me."

David

The work of Naomi Feil, dementia expert, author and developer of validation therapy is worth consulting. She gives valuable insights into the processes those with dementia go through to compensate as they lose certain faculties. Thus for example when short term memory fails, those with dementia will try to restore the balance in their lives by retrieving earlier memories. When they begin to lose their eyesight they will try to see with the mind's eye and when they can't hear what is happening around them anymore, they will listen to sounds from their past.

Deeply connecting

We have the opportunity to learn from those with dementia because they can teach us about our own humanity.

We can participate in ending the emotional isolation felt by those with dementia by being with that elder, and recognising that their need to give and receive love has not disappeared. When I visited my grandmother in the home where she was being nursed as her dementia progressed, all I could do was just be with her. Puzzled she would say to me, "I don't know who you are". I would reply, "It doesn't matter who I am, all that matters is I love you."

She would say "I don't know why I am so old and still alive" and I would explain, "You are letting go, piece by piece". "Is this dying?" she would ask. "It is difficult doing this dying. It's difficult living. I don't remember anything at all, nothing." I would try to encourage her, "I know but all you need to know is that I love you and I remember enough for both of us. You don't need to remember anything, all that matters is I love you."

"I Love You."

Communication is so much more than an exchange of information. It is the means by which we express our thoughts, feelings, hopes and dreams. It may be a glance, a touch of the hand, a hug, or a smile that connects us to another human being banishing loneliness and a sense of isolation.

"They invented hugs to let people know you love them without saying anything"

Bil Keane, comedian

We need not always fill the voids or silences with words. Patience and presence is the key when communicating and connecting emotionally with someone on their dementia journey.

"Mum just seems like an empty shell of a person now. I find it hard to remember that there is a beautiful pearl inside because her shell seems so difficult to open."

Maureen, carer

Understanding how to "open the shell" gives us opportunities to meaningfully connect with someone with dementia – even if only for a fleeting moment.

It is important for someone with dementia to receive reassurances and feel connected with familiar activities and people to create a sense of belonging, identity and connection.

Communication challenges

There may be specific challenges when attempting to communicate with an older person with dementia as they may have problems communicating their thoughts and feelings. There are many reasons for this. They may:

- not understand what you are saying to them, or know what is going on around them;
- confuse the past with the present reality;
- have problems remembering normal routines;
- have varying awareness levels;
- experience physical and social environment disorientation;
- have reduced insight and awareness of problems;
- have difficulties with memory recall;
- become slower at making conversation;

- repeat themselves;
- be unable to convey much information;
- say things that are not based on the reality of the listener;
- have difficulties reading or writing;
- make poor eye contact.

Adapted from guidance from the Alzheimer's Society 2009

BE AWARE

We can still relate to elders with dementia in emotionally meaningful, creative and dignified ways. Go with the flow of that person's commentary and stories and time frames. Allow yourself to loosen your moorings to the "present" to what is "real", to join with that person in their world and engage with their emotions and needs. By communicating with them with empathy you will help to reduce their stress, enhance their dignity and increase their happiness.

Tips for positive communication

Introduce yourself by your name
"Hello, it's me", can be confusing.

Exude a positive attitude
A person with dementia takes their cues from you so if you are smiling and upbeat chances are the elder will follow suit. Smiling is infectious.

Be complimentary
Most people tend to be in a better mood if you say something nice about them. Challenge yourself to find out what

it takes to make that elder's day, to help them feel good about themselves.

Talk about one thing at a time
Leave a time gap between any questions and rephrase their words back to them. Speak slowly to allow them time to understand. Look directly at them.

Listen actively
If you don't understand something politely let them know. Stay calm and relaxed and focused.

Enter their world
Enter their reality rather than argue with their facts, or correct inaccurate statements they may make.

Have patience
Give an elder extra time to process what you say. If you ask a question, give a moment to respond. Don't let frustration get the better of you when they repeat questions.

Understand there will be good days and bad days
People with dementia will have ups and downs just like anyone else.

Be aware of signs of distress
These may include looking around, fidgeting, walking away, mumbling.

Engage
Ask simple but positive and respectful questions such as "Do you have everything you need, what would you like me to explain?"

Break down tasks

Taking an individual through the steps of a task as it is performed will allow them to express themselves, highlight any anxieties and make them more comfortable.

Remind them

If necessary go over what has just happened, tell them what is happening now and what is about to happen. Use simple but clear language.

Keep eye contact

This is especially important before any personal care takes place.

Recognise pain

Some people with dementia are not able to adequately express pain or discomfort verbally, but you may be able to see a grimace or notice a sigh or groan. DO be prompt and maintain accurate delivery of pain medication, ensure you give the doses at the correct time to prevent break through pain.

Use non-verbal cues

For example, maintain eye contact and smile. This helps put an elder at ease and will facilitate understanding. Use touch, gestures, tone of voice and pointing as well as words – for example, show the person an object that relates to what you are saying. Mime simple tasks. Use sign language.

Observe

Watch the person's mood, breathing and movement. Listen to words and metaphors that may give clues to what they are trying to express. Learn to recognise and read their expressions.

Adapt and modify
Make sure activities are success orientated and failure free, enhancing the confidence of the elder.

Respond
Do not ignore an elder or their comments or complaints, if you can't answer a question try and find someone who can.

Use picture cards
These can help those with communication challenges.

Promote positive social encounters

Use life histories
Encourage relatives to bring in photographs showing important people, places, events and interests with explanatory notes and captions. Life histories provide opportunities to really get to know and engage with each individual as well as provide information for planning activities.

Use memories as medicine
Time travel to happy memories for that elder to help them escape from pain or anguish.

Practice mirroring techniques
Match and express their emotions back to them. You can speak back to them saying, "I see and feel you are angry/sad/happy". They will know they have your attention and a bond can be shared.

SING and use music
A person's ability to engage in music, particularly rhythm playing and singing, remains intact late into dementia. We can use

music to maintain relationships when we lose our words. I go into care homes and sing for and with relatives, staff and residents. Relatives have cried when they've told me they've sung with their parents. They say, "I got my mum back that day". These moments are so important to build upon and to cherish.

Validate

Don't ignore their emotions. Painful feelings that are expressed, acknowledged and validated by your attentive listening will diminish. Painful feelings that are ignored or suppressed will indeed increase. If you can engage with them with empathy and respect, those with dementia will feel listened to and supported. I highly recommend that you explore validation therapy and the book *The Validation Breakthrough*, written by Naomi Feil and now available in its third edition. Developed in the 1960s and 1970s by Naomi Feil, validation therapy for dementia offers empathetic holistic therapy. Some improvements this therapy may bring about in those with dementia include: displaying more social controls; less crying, pacing, and withdrawal; more verbal and non-verbal communication; and an improved sense of self-worth.

Remember

Everyone can be reached. We just need to find the right ways for that individual with love and perseverance and an open heart.

Understanding and coping with behavioural changes

All of us share the basic human needs for love, attachment, inclusion, comfort and identity. If these needs are not met our emotional and behavioural state will alter.

Remember

Interacting with a person who has dementia is all about feelings. In the early stages, these individuals often realise that something is wrong and may consequently be uncomfortable in interacting with others. There will be times when elders with dementia become agitated and aggressive and display other unwanted behaviours. Try to find out what is behind the behaviour. Is it sickness, sadness, environmental factors, fatigue, depression, or provocation?

Learning about the history, background and interests of each elder is essential to address challenging behaviours, and communication of this knowledge among carers is critical. All family members and staff need to be on the same page and communicate and share what they know about each resident. Everyone needs to know what triggers certain behaviours and try to avoid doing these things where possible. It is important to remember that the behaviour of those with dementia is not merely a function of physical changes in the brain but a reflection of physical, social and psychological events and changes that have occurred over that person's entire life span. Let's try to understand why we are encountering this behaviour, empathise and identify some positive actions and coping strategies.

Coping with confusion of time and place

Elders may make statements that indicate that they are confused. Examples are: "I want to go home!"; "This isn't my house"; "When are we leaving?" or "Why are we here?". Wanting to go home is one of the most common reactions for an Alzheimer's or dementia patient living in a care home. There's an emotional component to understand and empathise with.

"Often people are trying to go back to a place where they had more control in their lives."

Briony, carer

"We must translate some of the statements and questions such as: 'I want my mum'; 'I want to go home'; 'When is my bus?'; 'Where is my sister?'. The answer we give can make the person feel happy, content and comfortable or anxious, upset and lost. What does 'Mum' mean? It's comfort, a hug. Mums make things right, will sort things out for you. As a child you run out of school distressed and Mum will fight the world for you, when all seems wrong Mum makes it right. So we need to look at the person and see how we can make things right in their world now. 'I want to go home', might be hunger, needing the toilet or they just don't recognise their surroundings. If they ask 'Where is my sister?' and you respond with the name of her sister, 'Rosemary knows you are here, she has arranged this for you', they may say 'you know Rosemary?'. Straight away you have something in common to make them feel 'right'."

Mandi Randall-Cramp,
Sonnet Care Homes

Do

- Be patient and offer reassurance. Meet them positively in their own reality of "time travel". Try to understand their feelings and not make them feel as if they are "wrong".
- Offer simple explanations along with photos and other tangible reminders to help. Sometimes, however, it can be better to redirect the person and suggest an activity like going for a walk, or try getting a snack.

- Try to find a kind response if they ask specific but difficult questions such as "When are we leaving?". You might respond with, "We can't leave until later because .... the traffic is terrible / the forecast is saying there's bad weather / it's too late to leave tonight". Sometimes a *therapeutic lie* is needed, and is the kindest thing you can say in that situation, if telling the truth would cause pain, confusion, or mean they would not be safe.

Don't

- go into lengthy explanations or reasons, keep it simple.

"We had a resident who always thought that it was 1995 and she was forty years old. She would worry about the four dogs she used to have then. She fretted constantly, wondering whether the neighbour had remembered to walk them and feed them, and would get very anxious. We sometimes had a member of staff call her, pretending to be her neighbour, to tell her not to worry she was looking after them. Usually this would calm the resident. We even wrote her a note signed with the neighbour's name saying she had the dogs and all was well. The note worked to remind her and reassure her over and over again because she had such poor short term memory."

Susan, care home manager

READING TIP

Contented Dementia by Oliver James (Vermillion 2009) is a useful explanation of the Specialised Early Care for Alzheimer's (SPECAL) method which promotes a way of using the past to make sense of the present.

Coping with accusations

You may find that you are on the receiving end of false and unfounded accusations. Examples are, "You stole my jewellery" or "I have lost my watch, you have it!". This can occur in the early stages of dementia as brain cells deteriorate.

DO

- Ask them where they last saw the object, or ascertain if they have a favourite hiding place, and check wastepaper baskets and bins. Ensure your response can not be interpreted as accusatory or in any way doubtful of their competence as this could feel demeaning for the elder and escalate into anxiety and confrontation.
- Use validation therapy. For example, if an elder believes someone is stealing her wedding ring when in reality these items are being hidden by her you might respond in this way, "Your wedding ring is gone? Such a beautiful ring, I am sure you looked lovely on your wedding day. How did you and your husband meet?" thus diverting the conversation to something pleasurable and happy.

"I put the wedding ring on a chain around my neck for my mum and that stopped her getting anxious about where it was."

Tess, carer

CONSIDER

This experience of theft can be a mirror of deeper losses or previous experiences that may have caused suffering for that elder. Some careful unravelling may be required.

Coping with hallucinations

Hallucinations can be caused by changes in the brain which, if they occur at all, usually happen in the middle or later stages of dementia. Hallucinations can be visual for an elder with dementia but they can hear sounds that are not real and experience smells that are not there too.

"I was looking at the photos on the wall. I was frightened because the people in the photo were waving at me."

Eddie

"My hallucinations just jump at me. My therapist taught me to count tiles or flowers on the wallpaper. She called it distraction therapy."

Carol

"I kept smelling burning all the time."

Elaine

Do

- Speak calmly and kindly.
- Check the environment. Turn on lights so the room is well lit, turn off anything that might be triggering a hallucination such as a TV, or radio.
- Check for infection, dehydration and delirium.
- Check medications for side effects.
- Be aware that something as simple as deteriorating hearing and eyesight can contribute to any confusion, so ensure check-ups and assessments are done.
- Try distraction techniques. For example, if they're hearing voices that aren't there, try chatting to them. It's harder to hear voices, if someone is really talking to you.

- If they can 'see' someone, sit facing them and get eye contact if you can. If they can see you clearly during the hallucination it could make the experience less powerful and less intense.
- Acknowledge how they might be feeling during the hallucination. For example, "It sounds very scary, I can see how upset you are".
- Validate it, as it is very real for them. In fact, knowing you don't believe them might make them even more upset and anxious. Use validation techniques in talking to and comforting the elder, rather than telling them they are wrong. For example, if the elder thinks you are his wife who passed away five years earlier and he wants to take her back to their home, you could respond with, "You miss her and you want to be back in your house. What do you like doing there the most?"
- Have a meaningful conversation with that elder, by rephrasing the situation and reminiscing you can guide their experience more positively.
- Make sure you take some notes about the hallucinations. For example, how long they last, what they involve, what time of day they happen. Refer to details of any medication they might already be taking, which may be helpful for those who may wish to prescribe effective medication for the hallucinations if absolutely needed.

CONSIDER

Art or music therapy, reminiscence or pet therapy have helped older people cope with hallucinations and agitation. You could look at www. unforgettable.org.

Coping with aggressive outbursts

Mid to late stage dementia and Alzheimer's disease often present behavioural issues. The sadness, anger, paranoia, grief, confusion and fear that people with the disease experience can result in aggressive and sometimes violent speech or actions. Medication, especially for those with dementia, has been used historically to tackle behaviour including shouting, delusions and psychotic symptoms. Latest evidence suggests that powerful sedative drugs are used too early, and can have serious negative side effects. We need first to discover whether there is any underlying emotional distress to heal and work on releasing the source of agitation.

Statements such as "I want to go home", "I don't want to eat that", "I don't want a shower", or "I don't want to get dressed" can escalate into aggressive behaviour. Aggression may be coming from a place of fear, and anxiety. Those with dementia, in response to feeling overwhelmed or helpless, can resort to biting, hitting and kicking.

DO

- Make sure they aren't putting themselves (or anyone else) in danger.
- Remember in situations of verbal or physical aggression to try and identify the cause. Are they in physical or emotional pain or both? Are there environmental factors such as being in an unfamiliar situation, or communication difficulties and therefore frustration?
- Try to shift the focus to something else, speaking in a calm, reassuring manner. However sometimes trying to talk to someone and calm them down can serve to agitate them.

- Try to divert them with calming activities such as simple arts and crafts or untangling wool or fiddling with a bottle of coloured water, eating, simple gardening.
- Use the option of walking away and giving them some space if it seems appropriate.
- Consider using validation therapy and deeper forms of counselling, which can help address loss, bereavement and traumatic events. Past trauma can easily rise to the surface and may seem out of context to you as that elder moves between timeframes and memories.

Don't

- engage in an argument or force the issue that's creating the aggression;
- try to forcibly restrain the person unless there is absolutely no choice.

BE AWARE

There can be all sorts of factors from past and present contributing to aggression. Try not to take aggressive outbursts personally.

"The biggest way to stop aggressive behaviour is to remove the word no from your vocabulary!"

Peter, carer

Coping with risks of falls

As Alzheimer's progresses into middle and later stages, it causes a decline in muscle strength, walking and balance. Sometimes falls occur because of poor decision-making skills.

Some medications can increase the risk of falls. See www.
verywell.com.

"I kept trying to explain to my husband that he shouldn't get
out of his chair without my help. He is always falling but you
see he has been walking his whole life and just forgets he is
not strong enough or steady now. It's really sad."

Anita, carer

DO

- Check if they are in pain or uncomfortable. Be sure to
  evaluate this possibility, If pain is an issue, you may be
  able to alleviate it through a different position or some
  medication. See www.verywell.com.
- Remove loose mats and clutter.
- Consider marking edges of stairs with bright masking
  tape.
- Ensure there is a dimmer switch or nightlight for orientation and to reduce anxiety.
- Consider whether the older person may be getting up,
  even if too weak, because they are hungry or thirsty. Be
  sure to offer plenty to drink and eat so that this need is
  met. Ascertain if they need the toilet too.
- Consider whether boredom might be a factor. Is the
  person you care for just looking for something to do?
  Try to think of meaningful activities to share. **Please
  see How to Support Creativity and Activity section.**
- Explore whether loneliness could be a factor. Some
  people try to walk around by themselves when they're
  not able to because they are lonely. Social interaction
  is critical for people of all ages, and this need doesn't
  disappear when someone has dementia. Make sure

where possible that there are chances for socialising with others.

- Be aware that you could not only decrease the chance of falls, you could also help improve their overall mood and quality of life. See www.verywell.com.

See Fischer Center for Alzheimer's Research Foundation, People With Alzheimer's at High Risk of Falls and Injury, www.alzinfo.org.

Engage with relatives

Relatives hold the thread of continuity and are the bridge between worlds for those with dementia, so encourage them to help you understand why their relative might respond or behave in a certain way. They can provide you with historical information about the person who is coming into your care that can give you vital clues as to how to engage with and understand their needs. You need to have enough knowledge to be sensitive to important things like habits, the ways that person likes things to be done, and where they might need support. Help relatives to think about aspects of living that might make all the difference to their loved one in care and share their thoughts with you. Relatives can also share the emotional aspects of the move to a care setting, helping the elder settle more easily.

To understand their background and important aspects of their life discover:

- how they like to be addressed (first name, Mr, Dr, Miss etc.);
- their favourite drinks and food;

- clothing choices;
- preferred bedding and bedtime rituals;
- bathing routines;
- appearance preferences;
- companionship likes and dislikes, (male, female, pets, children);
- levels of ability;
- "touch" likes and dislikes;
- names of family and friends, family structure, pets;
- occupation (significant experiences in working life, awards etc.);
- important life events (births, deaths, marriages);
- important values, cultural, sexual, religious;
- social background;
- significant or special places;
- education, favourite subjects;
- skills and talents;
- fears and anxieties;
- likes, dislikes.

CONSIDER

It is vital to understand the life experience of an elder to support their individuality. Photographs, objects and ornaments are important visual and tactile symbols of someone's significant memories and achievements, especially for people with dementia. These "memory joggers" can assist their recall and sense of individuality. Encourage the placing and use of such mementoes with those in your care, seeking assistance from relatives when needed.

See *What do you See?* training pack by Amanda Waring and Rosemary Hurtley.

Understanding and supporting sensory challenges

Changes in senses can occur with those that have dementia. However you as a carer can help them live a positive life in spite of these challenges by aiding their awareness and acceptance and helping them adapt to the changes. To do this it will be helpful if you understand their experience and put into action some of the tips mentioned below.

VISUAL CHALLENGES

In some cases of dementia people you care for may have 20/20 vision but still experience problems seeing because the brain may not interpret the information properly.

"I did not think that getting a diagnosis affecting cognition would affect senses, so when I started to have sensory challenges I did not think it had anything to do with dementia."

Peter

"In shops they always have a big black mat and that looks like a hole, so it is perception and a leap of faith to actually step on to it."

Tommy

"Coming out of a shop, I find myself jumping (when I see a reflection of people in the silver doorframe) as if there is somebody there and I am trying to avoid them ... that's kind of frightening."

Alan

"Shopping is a nightmare now as I experience double vision and ghosting. Add sensory overload and it's all too much."

Agnes

Tips for supporting those with visual challenges

- Ensure an elder has clean and correct glasses.
- Ensure there is bright, even lighting (to reduce shadows).
- Encourage the use of talking books.
- Consider coloured overlays to help them read.
- Consider a white folding stick, if they will consent to it, to help with vision and perception and alert others to the visual challenges faced by that individual.
- Encourage access to opticians and orthoptists who could help with double vision. Ensure they know what type of dementia the individual has.
- Try approaching people from other organisations that can help, such as an RNIB locality officer or an NHS allied health professional.
- Be patient and allow the elder time to process.

HEARING CHALLENGES

Hypersensitivity to noise and certain tones, noisy environments and information overload can be of real concern to those with dementia.

"Noise in acute hospital wards can be a particular problem for people with dementia, increasing levels of anxiety, anger and distress and potentially affecting someone's appetite, sleep pattern and awareness of pain."

Shifting the Paradigm, NHS Lanarkshire guidelines

"My difficulty with loud noise has a huge impact in my life."

Helen

"Any loud noise and I hit the ceiling."

Joy

"Can't stand music in shops ... find myself getting very angry ... it was torture."

Peter

"In noisy environments I just can't think ... my brain shuts down."

Agnes

Tips for supporting those with hearing challenges

- Give time for an elder to hear what you are saying, allowing the individual to process the information and then think of an answer.
- Use reflective listening by repeating back what has just been said to you.
- Reduce sudden unexpected noise and sensory overload which may lead to confusion.
- Suggest ear plugs if appropriate and safe to reduce noise.
- Ensure hearing aids are on and at the correct setting.
- Make sure you have eye contact when speaking and use short clear sentences.
- Other help can be found from an NHS falls officer or an NHS allied health professional.

TOUCH, TASTE AND SMELL

Those with dementia can find they have changes around touch, taste and smell. Often they can't differentiate between hot or cold. Taste changes affect appetite and eating habits. Smells can be intense and overpowering or in some cases their sense of smell can decrease.

TOUCH

"I feel the cold more."

Liz

"I've become more touchy-feely now ... I hug people which I didn't do."

Wendy

"I poured boiling water over my hands instead of into a cup and didn't feel it."

Ross

Tip – fit special taps that judge temperature.

TASTE

"I can't smell what I am cooking ... I use my imagination."

Nina

"My taste has changed ... never liked coffee now I am mad about it."

Liz

"I used to take sugar but now I don't like it ... I also don't like salt. I used to enjoy a pint but not now."

Peter

"Everything is quite bland now so you don't want to eat."

Archie

Tip – serve food on a much larger plate so as not to appear overwhelming and make the food into small canapés.

SMELL

"I'm hungry but sometimes food just doesn't smell or taste right. I can't tell if food is bad so I eat chocolate instead. I go around sniffing myself as I think I smell bad ... I use a lot of perfume."

Agnes

Tip – show any dates of packets of food etc to reassure food is alright, taste it yourself as well. There are very good sensory deprivation tools to enable carers to feel what it is like to have certain impairments, thus increasing empathy and understanding.

Adapted with kind permission from Agnes Houston leaflet *Dementia Sensory Challenges*.

Dementia care at night

The impact of sleep disturbance is considerable for those with dementia and sadly increases their risk of mortality and need for medications. They are more likely to sleep during the day, and as a result their nutrition suffers because of missed meals and drinks. They may suffer with **Sundowners** syndrome.

This is where an older person may exhibit increased confusion, wandering, agitation, hallucinations and general disorientation from late afternoon onwards. As a carer you may find this unsettling and frustrating so you will need to keep patient, and follow the night time carer tips to make it through these episodes.

Care tips for Sundowner's syndrome

Not all of these ideas will work for everyone; through experimentation you may find the right formula for your situation.

- Create individual care plans for elder residents. These can be highly effective for communicating the night time needs of residents to other carers.
- Allow the older person to be exposed to light in the early morning to help set an internal clock.
- Daytime napping should be discouraged to help regulate the sleep cycle.
- Encourage exercise throughout the day to expend excess energy.
- Limit caffeine intake, particularly in the afternoon.
- When you sense agitation coming on, try giving a five-minute hand massage or just hand holding for a few minutes.
- Music or other sounds like ocean waves or singing birds can be calming.
- Interaction with a pet has also been known to calm agitation.
- The use of a bedside commode can be helpful as leaving the room to go to the toilet makes it harder to get back to sleep.
- Maintain a comfortable temperature in the bedroom;

extreme temperatures may disrupt sleep or prevent an older person from falling asleep.

- Minimise night time noise where possible in any care setting, the noise of buzzers, pagers and staff talking can be overwhelming.
- Install movement sensitive lighting so that the light will dim or go out once the elder has moved on.

Adapted from Alzheimer's Society website

Self-care tips for night time carers

Relatives worry about their loved one's sleep patterns and care at night but rarely meet the night time staff in a care setting. Consider putting up photos with the names of night time staff to help provide some connection with relatives and to allow the elders themselves to recognise you. Ensure the day time staff have your contact details so that relatives can call you if needs be. Sadly too often night time staff can feel overlooked in terms of support and training, ensure you are involved by addressing this with your manager and making sure you are invited to staff meetings and residents' and relatives' meetings. Your concerns must be heard, for you are caring for others at their most vulnerable if you are a night time carer and your role is of huge importance.

It is also vital that you take care of yourself. Being a night time carer can impact on your well-being, your home life can be affected and inadequate sleep suppresses the immune system, making one more susceptible to viruses.

Follow these hints and tips to help you adjust and keep healthy.

- Organise your sleep time well during the day, making sure friends and family help you get the sleep you need.
- Eat healthy food at regular times.
- Drink more water, limit caffeine.
- Wear loose clothes and shoes.
- Have regular health checks.
- Take gentle exercise.
- Get as much daylight as possible when you can.
- Be aware you may have problems with concentration, so take extra care when driving.

www.myhomelife.org.uk

Please also see the section on How to Care for Yourself and Prevent Burnout.

Dignity in dementia

The complex nature of the problem of preserving someone's dignity is highlighted in dementia care as I mention in my book *Heart of Care*. Professional and ethical paradoxes occur when those living with dementia can't continue to meet their essential needs. Research shows how important it is to balance the individual's freedom of choice even among those who are no longer capable of making sound choices, against the ethical duty to make sound choices on their behalf.

Dementia expert David Sheard reminds us that fostering dignity and choice means focusing on who the elder with dementia is NOW not who they once were. In practice this can mean supporting someone in a different reality; the person may be wearing clothes, making food choices, occupying themselves and seeking new relationships differently from the way they have done in the past. Trying to enforce a past reality or use our logic will not work if we are to be truly person centred in our approach. Families who see it as their role to maintain a person's past wishes can strongly resist the practices of person centred care, so skilfull negotiation and communication to enable working in partnership with families may be required. The input of relatives is important so it is vital to reach a clearly defined consensus. Relatives need gentle support and understanding. If they are supported they can better help you support their loved ones who are affected by dementia.

Remember

Appreciate yourself and the care and support you are giving an elder. Often there will be times when those you care for seem unresponsive or ungrateful even, due to their dementia. I thank you on their behalf, from the bottom of my heart. Please read the poem below when you feel undervalued.

Gratitude

I may be old,
I may be slow,
But you walk
alongside me.

When I won't talk
or cannot walk,
yet you still
reach out to me

Your patience and compassion
means such a lot and
My heart says thank you
even when my words cannot.

for your acts of kindness
serve as reminders
that I am not alone.

Amanda Waring

4

How to Care for Yourself
and Prevent Burnout

"I know God will never give me more than I can handle,
I just wish he didn't trust me so much."

Mother Theresa

I hope these important pages will inspire you to maintain your own emotional, physical and spiritual health, to recognise how much you are needed and to understand that you are as important as those you care for.

Carers need to develop compassion and try to relieve the suffering of others. However, to care for others means that we have to learn to care for, and have compassion for, ourselves too. Self-care, self-love and self-responsibility are important attributes to cultivate if we wish to continue in sound mental, emotional and physical health. Yet how often do we listen to our own needs or nurture our own body, mind and spirit? Our duty of self-care is of primary importance, but how often do we put ourselves first? We all need to be nourished, supported and motivated to give the best care that we can. In this chapter I show you ways to assess your risk levels and innovative ideas to relax and restore you when the going gets tough.

Are you at risk of burnout?

Do not underestimate the emotional and physical toll that caring for others can have on us. All of us can become overwhelmed and stressed by our work. It is rewarding but challenging, physically and emotionally. If the stress of caregiving is left unchecked, it can take a toll on your health, relationships and state of mind, eventually leading to burnout. If constant stress at work or home has left you feeling helpless, disillusioned and completely exhausted you may be suffering from burnout. Burnout is a state of emotional, mental and physical exhaustion caused by excessive and prolonged stress. When you're burned out, it's difficult to do anything, let alone look after someone else. When we neglect our own self-care, tiredness, depression and thoughtlessness can take hold. Thoughtless behaviour can then escalate into abuse, be it physical, or emotional. Too often breaches of dignity have occurred because burnt out staff have lost the ability to care or assess what is acceptable. Learning to recognise the signs of caregiver stress and burnout is the first step to dealing with the problem.

Common signs and symptoms of caregiver stress and burnout

- Anxiety, depression, becoming frustrated and irritated easily;
- feeling tired and drained most of the time;

- difficulty sleeping;
- overreacting to minor nuisances;
- new or worsening health problems;
- trouble concentrating;
- drinking, smoking, or eating more;
- neglecting responsibilities;
- cutting back on leisure activities;
- seeming to catch frequent colds.

Your emotional life can be affected in the following ways:

- you neglect your own needs, either because you're too busy or because you don't care anymore;
- your life revolves around being a carer, but it gives you little satisfaction;
- you have trouble relaxing, or switching off;
- you're increasingly impatient and irritable with the older people you're caring for;
- you feel helpless and hopeless and increasingly resentful;
- you withdraw from friends and social contacts, losing interest in work and life.

Actions for self-care and preventing burnout

Firstly invest in things outside of caregiving that give your life meaning and purpose, whether it's your family, your faith, or a favourite hobby.

Do

- Embrace your decision to become a carer.
  Acknowledge that, despite any resentments or burdens you feel, you have made a conscious choice to provide care to older people

or loved ones. Focus on the positive reasons behind that choice. Why did you become a carer, are there deep, meaningful motivations that can help sustain and renew you through difficult times. **What do you enjoy most about being a carer?**

- Focus on the things you can control.
- Enjoy your health, being in the sun, walking the dogs, hugging your children. **What can you focus on that brings you joy today?**
- Celebrate the small victories.

  If you start to feel discouraged, remind yourself that all your efforts matter. You don't have to cure an elder's illness to make a difference. Don't underestimate the importance of making that older person feel safe, comfortable, and valued. At the end of a person's life it won't be the medication or nice surroundings that matter but the love that they have received. Expressing love in care can restore the elder and the carer. **What victory, however small, can you celebrate today?**

- Find appreciation.

  Studies show that carers who feel appreciated experience greater physical and emotional health. Caregiving actually makes them happier and healthier, despite its demands. But what can you do if the person you're caring for is no longer able to feel or show their appreciation for your time and efforts? Try to imagine how, if not preoccupied with illness or pain (or disabled by dementia), he or she would feel about the dedicated care you're giving? Remind yourself that the person would express gratitude if he or she was able to. If working in a team, consider having a staff meeting where everyone says what they appreciate about each other's roles. **What is there to be grateful for today?**

- Appreciate your own efforts.

  If you're not getting external validation, find ways to acknowledge and reward yourself. Remind yourself of the good you're doing, the difference you are making to the lives of others.

Consider making a list of all the ways your caregiving is making a positive difference. Refer back to it when you start to feel low. **What can you appreciate about your caring today?**

- Talk to a supportive family member or friend.
  Positive reinforcement doesn't have to come from the elders you're caring for, or management. When you're feeling unappreciated, turn to friends and family who will listen to you and acknowledge your efforts. **Who can you talk with today?**
- Speak up and ask for help.
  Don't expect friends and family members to automatically know what you need or how you're feeling. Let them know and seek professional counselling if needed. The citizen's advice bureau can help. **Who do you love that you can reach out to today?**
- Say "yes" when someone offers help.
  Don't be shy about accepting help. Let friends/family co-workers feel good about supporting you. Share a list of small tasks that others could easily take care of, such as picking up your children, walking pets, making meals for the freezer. **Who can you say yes to today?**
- Be willing to give up some control.
  People will be less likely to help if you micromanage, give orders, or insist on doing things your way. So let your husband make the children's lunchbox! **Can you give up some control today?**
- Prioritise activities that bring you enjoyment.
  Make regular time for things that bring you happiness – dancing, music, the gym, working in the garden, seeing friends. Give yourself permission to rest and to do things that you enjoy on a daily basis. You will be a better carer for it. After a break/ rest, you should feel more energetic and re-focused and positive. **What has brought you joy today?**

- Find ways to pamper yourself.
  Small luxuries can go a long way towards relieving stress and boosting your spirits. Light candles and take a long bath. Ask a friend or partner for a massage. Get a manicure. Buy fresh flowers for the house. **What else might make you feel special?**

- Focus on one simple thing.
  By allowing yourself to focus on one thing at a time, a simple thing like hearing birdsong outside your window, the smell of fresh sheets as you fold them, you start to live in the present. This is a vital aspect of self-care. Slow down and BE. **What simple thing will you give your full attention to today?**

- Make yourself laugh.
  Laughter is an excellent antidote to stress and a little goes a long way. Read a funny book, watch a comedy, or call a friend who makes you laugh. **What made you laugh today?** *Share it.*

- Change your perspective.
  Feeling powerless is the number one contributor to burnout and depression. And it's an easy trap to fall into as a caregiver, especially if you feel helpless to change the situation. You may not be able to change circumstances but you can change the way you feel about things. Mindfulness apps such as headspace can help you relieve stress or you could try yoga, or deep breathing. Even a few minutes in the middle of an overwhelming day can help you feel calmer and bring a clearer perspective. **Can you try a five minute meditation today?**

- Take care of your body.
  Don't add to the stress of your caregiving work with avoidable health issues. We need our good health in order to thrive. **What have you done to keep yourself healthy today?**

- Exercise.
  When you're stressed and tired, the last thing you may feel

like doing is exercising BUT it is a powerful stress reliever and mood enhancer. Aim for 30 minutes where possible to boost your energy and help you fight fatigue. **Can you make time for exercise today?**

- Eat well.
  Nourish your body with fresh fruit, vegetables, whole grains, beans, lean protein, and healthy fats such as nuts and olive oil. These foods will fuel you with steady energy. **How healthy has your diet been today?**

- Keep hydrated.
  Dehydration causes tiredness, listlessness, irritation. This can lead to thoughtless behaviour, which can then lead to abuse, so it is vital that all staff are supported to keep their hydration levels topped up. This is especially important when working in over heated environments. Ensure water stations are available or the permission for bottled water is given. **How much water have you drunk today?**

- Get enough sleep.
  You need seven hours at least, when you get less, your mood, energy, productivity, and ability to handle stress will suffer. Avoid caffeine, listen to relaxation tapes or relaxing music before bed. LIMIT TIME ONLINE. Have a lavender oil bath. Wear earplugs. Snuggle with a hot water bottle or a loved one. **Can you go to bed earlier today?**

Are you at risk of compassion fatigue?

Compassion fatigue is what can happen when we witness the suffering of others, identify with it and empathise so much that we re-live their anguish and cannot let it go from our hearts and minds. As a carer you may be caring for elders in physical, mental and emotional pain, frequently hearing their cries and distress and tending to their fears and anxieties. The result may be that you experience compassion fatigue which is different from experiencing burnout.

Pioneering researcher in Post Traumatic Stress Disorder Dr Charles Figley is an American academic. Traumatology is only one of the many fields in which he is an expert. He has given a useful description of compassion fatigue. This is a state a person who is helping traumatised people may fall into where they become pre-occupied with those people re-experiencing traumatic events they have undergone. This can lead to symptoms of avoidance, numbing and persistent anxiety. It is easy to access Dr Figley's work online as he is prominent on a number of websites as well as having his own.

Dr Rachel Naomi Remen is another American academic who also has a significant presence online. She has done important work in the field of integrative medicine and has a website where she encourages people to explore healing together with her based on the essentially positive view that there is a hidden wholeness in everything and everyone. She has said however that we should not expect to remain untouched by exposure to suffering and loss on a daily basis. This would be unrealistic, like thinking we can "walk through water without getting wet".

Often the most caring carers, the most compassionate, are individuals who have gone through trauma in their own life or in fact received very little care or nurture themselves. Through becoming a carer they are redressing the balance. They may have great empathy but if caring for others triggers their own unaddressed difficult life experiences compassion fatigue can be the result.

When a carer experiences compassion fatigue and hopelessness then stress and a sense of inadequacy follow. Assess your own levels of susceptibility to compassion fatigue by honestly answering the questions below with a yes or no answer. If you answer yes to most please take pre-emptive action by following the exercises and advice in the rest of this chapter.

- I feel overwhelmed by the needs of others around me.
- I think I am affected by their suffering.
- I don't believe I can make a difference to them.
- I am a perfectionist.
- I can't let go of thoughts of someone's suffering.
- Their suffering becomes mine.
- I can't switch off at night without seeing their pain or sadness.
- I am not doing enough.
- I worry I might do or say the wrong thing.
- I have thoughts of my own death.

Ways to help compassion fatigue

Develop emotional strength and the courage to witness and endure stress
Some ways of doing this are to: take one step at a time, one day at a time; nurture humour; be able to grieve and let go. It is also important to develop the ability to reflect, value yourself and your time and make friends with yourself again.

Keep objective
Cultivate the ability to be non-judgemental and non-reactive to emotions directed to you as a carer. Elders may be angry through pain, spiteful through fear, critical through feeling a loss of control. Protect your boundaries and make it clear that you are there to help, but not to be verbally abused. Be clear that the motivation for such emotions may have nothing to do with you. Objectivity is the way to stay healthy.

Release Guilt

Guilt can play a terrible part in disturbing our well-being. If as a carer you know that you slipped up, made a mistake or showed frustration, forgive yourself and know that you have another day tomorrow to make this right and start again. Feeling guilty can be a self-defeating habit. Know that you deserve time to rest, to recharge your batteries and to reflect on how you will do things differently the next time.

Let go of the stress of others

You are not meant to carry the burdens of others for them at the expense of your own well-being, so at the end of the working day find ways to disconnect from your caring work. Often after a day of caring one can feel exhausted, not so much from the physical labour as from working in an environment that feels like emotional soup, where feelings expressed or not are heightened. This can tire most people. One care home manager bundles up all her cares and concerns and places them all in an imaginary bin bag which she then throws out of her car window at the nearest roundabout to her home! It works for her. Use what imagery might work for you.

Tips

- Wash your hands in salt water once home, or even have a bath in Himalayan pink salt. This helps clear your energy field from that of the other person. The salt contains properties that cleanse the parts that other soaps cannot reach! It works on an energetic level, and I recommend you try it.
- Burning incense can help clear you as can using frankincense oil on your wrists, feet and forehead.

- I will also burn "smudge" or cedar or white sage to clear myself and my home.
- Stand barefoot on the earth and feel stress and concerns moving through your feet, flowing out into the earth.
- An exercise that can be effective is imagining that you are wearing an invisible uniform of bright light during your working day. Imagine that this extra layer of light protection absorbs all the stress and upset, aggression, loneliness or despair that you may have encountered. In your mind's eye leave it outside when you get home, to be cleaned overnight, leaving you free to enter your space as you, without carrying everyone else's thoughts, anxieties, and grievances. You may find just the purposeful action of removing your work clothes allows you to leave work and cares behind.

Use the medicine of visualisation and meditation

Attachments and concerns regarding the elders we care for are understandable, and often come to the fore at night time, but it is important that you can disengage to have a restful sleep. I have devised a meditation which helps you to free yourself from feeling overburdened, supporting you to maintain positive boundaries so that you can let go of the stresses of others. Using meditation does not require any specific beliefs, it is simply a journey inwards. You may choose to record the meditation and play it back to yourself. Even reading it to yourself will have a positive effect. A meditation is also available as a track on my *I Am Near You* CD.

Find a comfy chair and a room where you will not be disturbed for five minutes.

"Allow yourself to get comfy, settled, give yourself permission for this time for you. Take a few moments to feel your feet connected to the earth. Try and allow extraneous sounds to fade into the background, let your thoughts drift away like clouds across a sky, just observe them without becoming attached to them . . .. Breathe deeply and with each deep breath allow yourself to let go of some of the busyness of your life, affirm that for the next few minutes you will give yourself space to BE. Nothing to do, say, fix, change or worry about, this is your time to rest, restore and revive yourself. You deserve this time to feel relaxed. Take an even deeper breath and this time let it out with a gentle sigh, allowing yourself to let go that bit more.

Now imagine in your mind's eye that you are sitting on a soft rug on a grassy bank next to a beautiful calm lake on a summer's morning. You feel the warmth of the sun on your skin as you watch the dance of sunlight shimmering on the lake. You breathe in deeply the clean air as you take in the exquisitely beautiful surroundings – the willow trees dipping their fronds into the cool sparkling water, elegant swans gently weaving their way across the lake. You see the tall reeds fringing the lake swaying in the gentle breeze and watch the brightly coloured butterflies that play amongst them. You sit peacefully and happily savouring the beauty of your surroundings, listening to the delightful birdsong that serenades you, feeling content and safe, relaxed and rested.

You become aware of a delightful scent that reaches you and on the lake you see pink lotus flowers gently opening and releasing their fragrance, which you inhale deeply. You are happy and content savouring the exquisite aroma and breathing out any tension in your body. You are grateful that you have taken this time to just BE as you feel your heart opening just like the lotus flowers, and as your heart opens you are aware of a beautiful golden light that emanates from your heart surrounding you in a beautiful golden bubble, a bubble ▶

of unconditional love that nurtures you. You feel safe and happy within this golden bubble of light. You feel held, hopeful and restored within this golden heart light.

In this peaceful state you become aware of small sailing boats on the lake and in each one are those that you care for, they too are in their own individual bubbles of golden heart light. They steer their own boat/boats closer towards you, you can see their faces clearly – they smile and acknowledge you within your own heart light, and you are aware of their contentment, and their ability to steer their own boat so easily and happily navigate the lake. You feel that loving compassion between you and as the breeze picks up you see each person you care for enjoying the freedom and independence of sailing their own boat, you watch them with compassionate detachment as they sail further away from you. You see them just on the horizon, receding into the distance as you know that they are safe and protected within their golden bubbles steering their own ships and you feel at peace within your own bubble of golden light, knowing that all is well. You take a deep breath and realise how good it feels to be beside this lake in your golden heart space where there is nothing to do but just be, and as you allow yourself to be that gives others permission to do the same, to be free. You recognise that you can return to this lake and be with yourself any time you choose but for now you can bring yourself back to the present moment, the present time ... so ... very gently become aware of the sounds of the room, feel the chair that you are sitting on, stretch your fingers, ease your neck, return to your body. Stretch and take a deep breath in and a long breath out, become aware of your surroundings, run your hands through your hair, feel your feet, come back to the here and now. Recognise that meditations like these can help you when you feel overwhelmed by the needs of others. Realise how important it is to connect to our own life, our own heart and soul.

Remember

YOU ARE AS IMPORTANT AS THOSE YOU CARE FOR.

To give nurture means being nurtured. Please care for yourself emotionally, physically and spiritually so that there can be something left to give others! How can you place yourself at the heart of your own care? To do this, make a personal pledge. Write it down and place it where you and your loved ones can see it often. **To place myself at the heart of my own care I will:**

- set and maintain appropriate boundaries;
- attend to my physical and emotional health;
- make time for my personal life;
- keep a gratitude journal and count my blessings;
- reach out to the people I love;
- find ways to acknowledge loss and grief;
- allow myself to cry;
- have quiet time alone to relax;
- be out in nature or wherever I feel inspired.

Add any other promises to yourself that can support you and help you keep balanced.

Keep your candle lit

Taking time out in the form of meditation can be so beneficial. Meditation does not require any specific beliefs but it can help keep us peaceful and positive and resilient. This exercise can be done in two minutes and helps to significantly restore hope and peace. Allow yourself to focus on your heart, where we carry so much grief and stress. Imagine placing a candle within your heart, lit with a beautiful golden flame, focus on that flame in your heart, keep bringing your focus back to that golden flame within. Breathe with that flame, and when you are ready open your eyes and connect to your surroundings once more. Check in with yourself often to see if your candle is still lit. If it has gone out, with a thought of intent light it again. Sometimes I may need to light my heart candle ten times a day but each time I do I feel the calmness and compassion that comes from tending to my inner flame.

Prayer and connection

Finding a connection to a higher power, which provides a source of benevolence, comfort and empowerment may greatly enhance one's coping ability. When you feel overwhelmed say to whatever /whoever your faith dictates, "I surrender this to God/Jesus/Mother Earth/the Angels/Buddha/a higher power/the Christ within, and I go free". Hand your problems over and be willing to receive divine help.

Perhaps you might consider saying this serenity prayer to yourself when you feel overwhelmed with the pressure of caring for others. "God give me the serenity to accept the things I cannot change, the courage to change the things I can, and the wisdom to know the difference." The prayer was written by the American theologian, Reinhold Niebuhr.

Keep on keeping on

Struggle, sacrifice and responsibility are horrible ways to motivate oneself. Do not try to value success in outcomes so much that you ignore the process of your journey. If you have lost your passion or focus to "keep on keeping on" try and find people who inspire you and can re-inspire you with their passion and persistence. These may be co-workers, or people from history or fiction. Try and find your heroes to help you find the hero in you.

I love to quote the following story about Sir Winston Churchill, who at the age of 80, was asked to address the Oxford Student Union. He stood on the stage and spoke to the eager students, "NEVER GIVE UP". There was a pause before he looked the students in the eyes again and repeated, "NEVER GIVE UP". Another minute passed as he looked them more deeply in the eyes and then finally said, "NEVER GIVE UP". And with that he left the stage but his impact was huge. I think of this when I feel close to giving in, giving up and hiding under a blanket!

Another heroine of mine is Helen Keller who is famous for overcoming the misfortune of being both deaf and blind to become a leading humanitarian of the 20th Century. "I am only one, but still I am one, I cannot do everything but still I can do something, I will not refuse to do the something I can do."

Martin Luther King, the leading civil rights activist inspires me. "We must accept finite disappointment, but never lose infinite hope."

The medicine of creativity

Consider using your creativity to help you through challenging times. Paint, sing, write, dance out your frustrations or grief. I write poetry to help me move through darker times, those "what is the point" times. My poems then become positive mantras that I use and share as personal reminders to restore hope and self-belief and to recognise the value of our care, seen and unseen.

"If you plant a seed
and it takes root elsewhere,
don't turn your back
the seed is still there.
It's sowing that matters,
the courage to try.
Nerves may be shattered but the seed cannot die."

Amanda Waring 2001

Self-compassion

We may often be compassionate with others, but with ourselves it can be a very different story. Learn to be tender with yourself. We all want to feel loved but rarely take the time to acknowledge the parts of ourselves that feel unworthy of being loved. Try and soothe, forgive and comfort the deepest wounds you have. Be gentle, be kind, be patient, be compassionate with yourself and let your healing process begin.

"I keep myself at the heart of my own care to allow greater care of others."

Amanda Waring

5

How to Support Emotional and Spiritual Needs

"The three most important things in life are
to be kind, be kind, be kind."

Mother Theresa

For you as a carer to understand how to support the emotional
and spiritual needs of those in your care will be so valuable
and rewarding. You have the opportunity to help people in
a heartfelt way. Good emotional care is as vital as good medical practice. In old age whatever our faith, or lack of it, the
human need to put things in order, forgive, be listened to, feel
safe, find peace, acceptance, hope and understanding becomes
especially important.

Spiritual care is not solely about religious beliefs and practices, it is not a specialist activity or the sole responsibility of
the chaplain or faith leader, but it is about being open enough
to meet people's deepest needs. Spirituality may be a personal

but important part of an older person's journey from "doing" to "being". The simplest definition of spirituality is that aspect of us that gives meaning and purpose to life. It is about being connected with Creation, God, Buddha, a higher power, Great Spirit, the workings of the universe as well as ourselves and our feelings, and being connected to others.

"Spiritual care begins with encouraging human contact in compassionate relationship, and moves in whatever direction needs require."

NHS Education Scotland Guidelines

Discovering spiritual needs

It is important that an older person's spiritual needs are identified and valued as an integral part of their quality of life. When working alongside an elder, it is worth gently trying to ascertain the answers to the following questions.

- What faith if any provides support for them when the going gets tough? How can you provide easier access to religious texts or music?
- Does prayer or meditation help, or writing worries down? How may you facilitate this by providing a quiet space, or pads and pens?
- What friend, family member, staff member or religious figure would they like to consult with when they feel overwhelmed? How can you ease their lines of communication to these people?
- What has helped them cope or endure in past difficult experiences? How can you provide these solutions? It may be something as simple as a bath, a cup of tea, listening to Mozart, stroking an animal, sleeping, being hugged etc. . . .

Heartfelt listening

Heartfelt active listening is a powerful tool to support the emotional and spiritual needs of others. Having regrets, loss, unresolved difficulties or relationships can be a legitimate source of stress. Some older people may want to reflect on these with you. You can help by listening, without trying to fix anything or change the situation, but just receive the words of the older person who may then in their own mind be able to resolve the conflict or to accept it. When you listen from the heart it is amazing how much more you will remember and have empathy for the emotion of that person. Sometimes all we need is to be fully present in a situation. This benefits those we care for, but also releases us from outside interference which can prevent us from giving the quality of heartfelt compassionate care we wish to give.

Emotional support for transitions

As carers we need to give time, patience, compassion and understanding to ease transitions. Moving into a care home is often done at a time of crisis, following an illness, hospitalisation, the death of a partner/carer, so there are already strong emotional challenges present. The impact of moving into a care home on each older person will vary, but it will still be a massive upheaval and a major life event whatever the circumstances. Change can affect people's physical, mental, and emotional equilibrium. Moving into a care setting means an elder not only has to settle in but also fit in with other residents too.

We must understand the anxieties of someone who is unsure whether they are moving into a community of emotional support or spending the rest of their days in an institutionalised environment. We should realise an elder can feel bereaved, away from loved ones, their home, possessions, their pets, and fear the loss of independence and control over their life.

How you can help

- Welcome them warmly into their new environment. That first welcome will make all the difference to them feeling wanted and being part of the family of their new home, a place where they will possibly be for the rest of their days.
- Help them to personalise their rooms and use life stories to discover more about them.
- Create a neighbourhood of friends for them by seeking out like-minded residents and staff.
- Help them become familiar with the care home, its layout and routines, affirming, reminding and encouraging them all the while.
- Ensure outside areas are accessible and enjoyed where possible to help the settling in process and to provide a sense of place.
- Introduce them to night time staff who may be caring for them when they feel at their most vulnerable.
- Encourage relatives and friends to continue to visit and be involved in the home and share their knowledge of their loved one.
- Help them contribute to decision making aspects in the home, this is THEIR HOME after all now.

BE AWARE

A few phone calls to the relatives in the first weeks of the move sharing how their loved one is settling in will make a world of difference.

Making things better

When I ask carers what they do when they are stressed, or have had a bad day, how do they make themselves feel better, answers include: phoning a friend, going shopping, walking the dog, a hot bath, a glass of wine, playing with their children, hugging their husband, running, getting a massage, going to the cinema. Then I ask them whether they have discovered what made the elders in their care feel better "in the outside world". What brought that elder comfort and what freedom does the elder now have to do or have what brought them support? I continue by explaining that it is imperative we find ways, however small, to address fulfilling the criteria of each individual's "emotional medicine". All too often this information is missed out in care plans or interactions. I am not talking about likes or dislikes here but what was an emotional balm for the older person and could be again in some ways. We know an older person will face pain and loss and loneliness, so let's do what we can to help.

Find out

- What piece of music lifts their spirit? Can you have this accessible on an iPlayer? Can you listen to it and appreciate it together?

- What their favourite scent or smell is. They might find lavender, rose, or honeysuckle uplifting. Could you use a scented pillow spray or room spray to help them when they feel down? Small personal things make a big difference.
- Whether they used to like walking in natural settings. Can you bring in pinecones for them to hold, or their favourite flowers? Perhaps you could play a CD of sounds of the forest.
- What TV programme did they like, what comedy made them laugh? Can you access copies?
- If they are missing a husband or wife who can't be with them. If they can be reached can you make sure a greeting can be sent to be played often on an iPlayer? Or perhaps face time moments could be arranged, as well as encouraging visits.
- If an elder used to like to walk by the sea when they were unhappy. Can you bring in a bowl of sand for them to run their hands through, or play a CD of the sounds of the sea?

Create an inspired action plan, a spiritual recipe if you like, for each elder you care for. These details of what will provide comfort should be expressed meaningfully in the care plan as ways to promote the emotional and spiritual well-being of that person.

Understanding the importance of feeling needed

Do not ignore the emotional benefits for an elder of feeling needed. Having purpose and a sense of achievement is necessary for people to continue to thrive spiritually. Find ways you can provide opportunities for older people to contribute or to "give care" to others, (no slave labour!). Folding clothes, choosing flower arrangements, laying the table, reading to others, singing, welcoming others into the dining room could all be ways of including them and giving them a sense of being useful.

Emotional and spiritual care is a two way process that allows the elders to share with and minister to us too, through their words and insights and actions.

Mrs Jameson, an 86 year old carehome resident, said to me, "Now I am in this care home I can't get used to not being busy anymore or wanted. In my road", she said, "I was always the one people would come to first for baby-sitting, dog walking, cake sales and such. I just don't see the point of me anymore. I knew everyone on my street, I don't know anyone here. I am tired all the time and I can't bear it. The morning staff are so noisy, they wake me up every time they arrive."

I gently suggested that Mrs Jameson set her alarm and actually get up before the morning staff arrived, in order to welcome them in like a commissionaire. She looked a little suspiciously at me, but she tried it and loved it. She had found a role, a purpose. Staff really appreciated being welcomed to work in this way and Mrs Jameson felt that she had a responsibility to welcome them into "her home". This also reminded staff that the care home was her HOME as well as that of the other residents, something that can get forgotten in the busyness of care. Mrs Jameson got to know members of staff and they her and despite the early start Mrs Jameson's energy levels improved!

Adapted from *Heart of Care* by Amanda Waring

Tips to provide further emotional support

You can help those you care for to maintain their emotional health by:

- encouraging elders to enjoy life by using existing abilities;
- encouraging sharing of emotions, feelings, hopes and fears;
- supporting the inner values and beliefs that help people cope;
- building relationships, knowing the elders well enough to provide a varied and interesting day;
- recognising the themes, symbols, religious cultures that are important to people in your care;
- knowing your own strengths and limitations;
- being aware that when it is appropriate you can refer to another source of support such as as chaplain, counsellor, family member or friend.

Remember

Pay attention to your own emotional and spiritual needs. If you feel out of your depth seek help from someone you trust, or contact interfaith ministers or other support networks.

Providing spiritual and faith support

It is never right to impose your own beliefs and values on another, nor to try and convert anyone to your own faith. An elder should be enabled to express their faith in the way they choose. If the older person has a specific faith or spiritual beliefs find time to read to them, or together, passages from the holy books of their belief system.

Find favourite verses or prayers
Some people with dementia have certain verses and prayers
they've committed to memory and used throughout their life.
In a world of confusion, memory loss, or difficulty finding the
exact words, the practice of prayer can transcend some of those
cognitive losses. See www.verywell.com.

Observe Traditions and Rituals
Ensure an older person can participate in any religious services they may wish, whether in person or through watching
on TV, or listening to the radio or an iPlayer. Some people
with dementia might enjoy the familiar routine of a religious
service. For others, the stimulation and larger group of people
might make them anxious. Over the course of a year there are
several holy celebrations and events for many different faiths.
If possible, and where appropriate, involve the elders in commemorating those special times.

Use Touchstones
The tactile experience of holding something meaningful in
your hands can be powerful. Holding a necklace that has a
symbol of faith attached to it or a sacred book may be meaningful for some people, as may a polished stone with the word
peace written upon it. Find some significant objects of faith
that could be of comfort for those you care for. A precious
gift from a grandchild, or a cuddly toy that has meaning can
work equally as well.

The power of gratitude

You may encounter various states of depression in yourself
and in those you care for but a balm for those dark times that
is drug free and cost free is the practice of deep gratitude.

Developing gratitude inspires an ability to see the world through fresh eyes, to be appreciative and to value the positive aspects of ourselves, our colleagues and those we care for. So consider sharing one small thing that you feel you can be grateful for today with an elder and ask them to do the same. This could range from a cup of tea to the flowers by your bedside, a smile, or the planet itself. Doing the exercise could be nourishing for you both and allow deeper opportunities to connect and support each other too. You may even want to consider starting a gratitude circle once a week in your care setting where people come together to share with each other the things for which they feel grateful. It can be powerfully nourishing hearing the words of others and reminding ourselves of how much we can give thanks.

Provide an emotional care box

Loneliness, boredom and a sense of helplessness can overcome the human spirit, especially for those who are frail, enduring pain or chronic illnesses. When elders are unhappy or distressed a good way to help support them and assist all staff and relatives to reach out to them is by giving them easy access to an "emotional care box". This is a box or trunk within which can be an assortment of things to help the well-being of another. There should be one in each unit, or on every floor of a home. Items can be personalised and anything can be added that you feel would provide comfort and solace. Always replace what is used.

Examples of the kind of thing that can be put in such a care box are:

- soothing hand lotion, for hand massages;
- a CD player/iPod and a collection of relaxing music, sounds of the sea, birds etc.;
- a warm super soft blanket;
- cuddly toys;
- a collection of different fragrances;
- strokeable material e.g. velvet that is soothing to hold;
- uplifting colouring books and pens;
- a collection of inspiring, uplifting poetry;
- humorous verse;
- a Bible, a Koran, other multi faith religious books;
- self-help books;
- travel journals;
- prayer beads;
- photos of angels, saints, buddha;
- comedy audio recordings;
- a weighted blanket, wrap or lap pad.

The benefits of weighted blankets

Weighted blankets, wraps or lap pads are positive drug free options used to alleviate distress with those who have autism, but also work exceptionally well in elder care with those with dementia. A weighted blanket or weighted jacket is a safe and effective therapeutic solution, calming the body and helping aid a peaceful night's sleep too. Deep pressure touch helps the body relax, almost like a firm hug enabling someone to feel secure, grounded and safe. They can help calm restless legs and many other symptoms associated with those who are agitated, aiding Alzheimer's and Parkinson's disease patients.

You might be able to make your own as a joint project within the care home, as a productive, constructive activity.

There are instructions on youtube. They are also easy to purchase.

The medicine of kindness

Kindness in caring is without doubt an essential gift to share.

EXERCISE

Consider what values as a carer you may need to help you support the emotional and spiritual care of others. To help you identify your values, consider the following list to see which ones resonate most with you; acceptance, appreciation, balance, benevolence, clarity, centredness, commitment, compassion, co-operation, courage, dependability, dignity, enthusiasm, forgiveness, flexibility, generosity, gratitude, honesty, hope, humour, inspiration, integrity, kindness, love, loyalty, openness, patience, peace, practicality, respect, responsibility, tolerance, trust, wisdom.

Try to discover the values of those you care for too, as they reveal so much about a person, and during times of crisis or stress we can help remind each other to remain true to our values.

Adapted from *Heart of Care* by Amanda Waring

Checklist for promoting spiritual and emotional well being

- help them to develop their imagination and creativity and to continue learning new things;
- help them to keep and develop their sense of humour;
- help them to have something to look forward to, however small or unexpected;

- help them to feel that they belong and their participation is valued;
- help them to feel needed;
- help them to express their feelings;
- help them to nurture hope;
- help them to find peace;
- help them to feel loved and that their life has been worthwhile.

Remember

We all make a difference, no matter how large or small, it is sowing the seeds of dignity and compassion that matter and having the courage to try.

6

How to Support Creativity and Activity

"It is neither wealth or splendour, but tranquility and
occupation which give happiness."

Thomas Jefferson

I hope you will enjoy putting creativity and activity at the heart of your caregiving. Giving voice to our unique creativity provides us with a freedom of expression and a sense of purpose or delight that makes us feel alive no matter what our age. We all need a variety of activities in our lives from daily living tasks to well established hobbies to give us a sense of achievement and to be able to thrive emotionally, physically and spiritually.

Purposeful activities in elder care provide a structure to the day and can give a sense of belonging. Many older people can feel disconnected from significant people and routines, from their family or familiar surroundings, but activities such as music, art, gardening, or walking can restore interest and friendships. Activities can reduce restlessness and agitation and have health benefits by raising a person's mood, improving socialisation and preventing dependency.

An older person who is vulnerable or frail may have few expectations, their self-belief and sense of identity may be diminished, but being encouraged in small ways to participate using their remaining abilities restores hope and self-esteem. Being able to continue to contribute, to share with others, to give and to receive love can help people to find peace and dignity in old age. Sharing tasks and activities is a good way to bond.

It is important to get a balance between giving the right level of support and "taking over". Assessing what an elder can do is essential for a person-centred quality of life plan. Realise that this could change on a daily basis due to low mood or physical discomfort, be spontaneous and flexible in your approach and remember the changes in capability that will occur when someone has dementia.

Getting to know you

To help you find out what an older person needs to improve their social, emotional and creative health please try using the checklist below.

- What kind of life roles have they enjoyed? How can they be encouraged to maintain a role in ways that are important to them in their current community?
- What have they enjoyed in the past, what are their passions?
- What might they like to do to provide continuity with the past and engagement in the present?

- What levels of assistance do they need to follow through an activity?
- What attention span do they have to sustain interest and concentration?
- Do they like company, and if so how much?
- Do they prefer to spend time alone?
- Are they a morning or an evening person, when does their energy dip?
- Tailor activities to work with their time frames and energy levels.

Taken from *What do you See?* training pack by Amanda Waring and Rosemary Hurtley

Remember

Although some people may benefit from being connected with a former interest, others may not wish to do what they did before – their abilities and preferences may have changed or it may be too painful to be reminded of an activity that they used to do with friends and family. A sensitive approach is required. *Never force or bully someone into being involved with an activity.* Recognise individual choice. Some people are happy to sit and watch what is going on around them rather than be actively involved, but it is important to assess if sitting and watching is what they really want. If they are saying "No" to an activity try and think of another way to engage their interest if you feel that perhaps they really would rather be more involved. Pay attention to choice and consent and seek advice if unsure.

Keep on moving

It's important to encourage active exercise because sitting for long periods can hasten physical decline, causing severe problems in the care of the elderly. Muscles can waste, joints contract, leading to increased risk of fractures, heart and respiratory problems and bed sores. Inactivity can cause weight gain, continence difficulties, hostility, impatience and sleep disturbances. But physical activity has a positive effect on mood and mental alertness, and can improve flexibility, strength, and balance, relieve depression, aches and pains, and sleep disorders, and reduce agitation, confusion and memory problems.

So encourage and maximise every opportunity for an elder to move as much as possible. Try nature walks, gentle gardening, competitive physical games, walking netball, armchair dance, painting to music, drumming, yoga, or mini golf. With those with dementia it is important to encourage purposeful movement, such as cleaning, dusting, sorting, and washing. Tapping into someone's muscle memory with daily living tasks will assist in meeting their need to feel valued and purposeful. Get creative with the plan of action, discussing and making choices as a team effort with the older person. The wrong activity, or not enough to do, can have a damaging effect on an elder's health and well-being.

Sharing ideas

Remember, older people can still learn new things! If there is an activity you enjoy don't be afraid to offer to share that with an elder. Integrate technology into activities. Using a tablet, experience a video game together, or explore a virtual walk to one of their favourite places on google maps. Activities should not be stuck in a time warp. Share something of yourself with an elder and enjoy the journey of discovering activities together and exploring a variety of interests that could be:

- energising, energetic e.g. ball games, skittles, dance;
- peaceful, gentle e.g. meditation, yoga, colouring, boules;
- done alone e.g. crosswords, patience, solitaire;
- a mental challenge e.g. quizzes, debates, memory games;
- involving the senses e.g. baking, smelling herbs or spices, stroking pets, flower arranging;
- something completely new e.g. learning Italian, making sushi;
- social activities e.g. singing, wine tastings, tea parties;
- spiritual activities e.g. hymns, candle making, readings;
- encouraging communication e.g. storytelling, mime, writing;
- cultural e.g. poetry, art history, travel books;
- creative e.g. painting, pottery, sand art, woodwork, photography.

CONSIDER

Solitude is a normal human need and there can be too much emphasis on being "social". The elders you care for may be introverts who enjoy being in their bedrooms and do not often pursue interaction with others. They engage with life in fundamentally different ways to their extrovert counterparts. Activities for them might include birdwatching (invest in some binoculars), mindful colouring books, learning digital photography on line, making a collage, keeping a budgie, watching movies, writing a diary or journal, or listening to audio books. As a way of engaging with others they might enjoy baking cakes and biscuits for everyone.

Keeping motivated

Having a goal they can aim for is one thing that may motivate people. Consider using score cards, reward stickers, or commitment cards to monitor progress. Sharing and keeping an eye on each other's goals can be motivating too. Try to encourage people to use their abilities and not let issues of speed or time prevent them helping and contributing in some way. Plan with older people the type of projects they might like to engage in or make or teach. Share your own goals with the people in your care so that you can support each other. Provide opportunities for the elders to share their skills to enrich your life and deepen your relationship. Enjoy the process.

Remember

Keeping motivated and purposeful with activities means ensuring that whatever is being created – cards, knitting, embroidery, biscuits – can often have an end purpose as gifts for others, or as a charity fundraiser, or even to break the odd world record!

People feel inspired when united with a common cause, knowing that their creative output has meaning and a positive end result for others. This helps the elders feel connected to the wider world, knowing that they have made a difference and their contribution is needed.

Let elders know of, and have access to, online petitions and campaigns so that again their point of view can be registered and their influence felt in the wider community. You could try the campaigning communities of 38degrees.com or Avaaz.com.

Think outside the box

Do use the element of surprise and provide unexpected "happenings". Try something completely new:

- Learn Japanese, see the free language website www. duolingo.com.
- Try karaoke.
- Try different video games, wii fit, wii sports, puzzle and brain apps on iPads or Android tablets. Technology offers easy, fun ways to play games like Sudoku and Scrabble, or do crossword puzzles, through apps and websites accessed on tablets. Not only do digital games let elders magnify screens to see better and prevent eye strain, but they also do not require the dexterity needed to hold a pen or small pieces as physical games may do.
- Try learning magic tricks which can help with agility of mind and body and also entertain others.
- Have skype or face time lectures with guest speakers such as animal specialists who can show and tell animal stories, historians who can share stories and pictures, master cooks or gardeners who can share tips and memories.
- Try life drawing classes, calligraphy, chocolate tastings, learning the ukulele, belly dancing, musical recital, the art of bonsai, bee keeping, stand-up comedy. Unleash creative possibilities.

I recommend you try the websites of www.brightcopperkettles.co.uk and www.goldencarers.com. These have lots more inspiring ideas for you to draw from.

Promoting well-being in dementia

Activating wellness in dementia requires you as a carer to be playful and emotionally in tune. A sense of fun and spontaneity and joining in the moment are gifts that can change the atmosphere and lift the spirits. Work with the senses in a therapeutic way. Consider the themes and interests that are most evident in the lives of those you care for and place themed sets of memorabilia along shelves, corridors, and window sills to promote memories and interaction, bringing the richness and variety of the wider world into their personal space.

There are many activities that can be planned or spontaneous including art, music sessions, drumming circles, knit and natter groups, cooking, games, social events, reminiscence groups, exercise sessions, outings, special events, computer sessions or themed days.

"Working with dementia there is no 'right' way when it comes to activities, and no day is ever the same, just like our residents. Everyone is an individual no matter how old they are or at which stage of dementia they are. Before even considering introducing activities it is important to gather as much information as possible about the individual. This can be done by simply talking to them, building up trust, asking relatives and reading their care plan. Whilst it is important to find out all you can about the person it also helps if you share things about yourself too. Tell them about your children, holidays, pets, this helps to build up a mutual trust.

As and when possible allow the residents to be involved in activity planning. I always give options of what we can do or where we will be going on our regular minibus outings, but also be prepared to change this at any time to suit their needs. I have found that a lot of our residents in the early stages of dementia are reluctant to participate in 'group activities' as they can find this demeaning so instead of asking them to join in I ask for their help. Everyone needs to feel a sense of self-worth and to feel useful. We had an older lady Kate who would not come out on a minibus outing with others who had more progressed dementia as she felt demoralised but when she was asked to come along and help me she suddenly had a purpose and at the same time enjoyed the outing."

**Jo Whitehouse, Head of Activities,
Sonnet Care Homes**

Sharing meaningful activities with those with dementia

Often meaning is tied to past occupations or hobbies, so if you don't know the person's history, ask their family members or observe their reaction to different activities. If they are distressed or uncomfortable in any way discontinue that activity and note the ones to which they have responded well.

Activities for men

In these changing times of gender equality it is still important to remember the times and roles that elders experienced, whilst of course allowing for personal choice in exploration of traditional male and female activities. You may find that men may not care for the activities that women enjoy, or indeed, at times, want to be involved in activities with women. So provide social opportunities for men to be with other men, to build friendships, mentorships and discuss what matters to them or makes them laugh. Consider running a men's group, seek out men in the community, family members, or male staff to join in discussions and sharing, perhaps using, themes. Try and match those with similar interests, military men to discuss the war, farmers, or business men to discuss the joys and challenges of past occupations. Utilise the past occupations of others to benefit the care setting or home. It is good to be needed and employed meaningfully. Especially if men gained pleasure from doing odd jobs around the house, find out whether they could help with chores like fixing bird tables, putting fuses in plugs, hanging pictures, rubbing down furniture, polishing silver, or painting shelves. These are all small helpful tasks to aid the community and promote self-esteem. You may want to consider setting up a men's games night using strategic games such as chess, poker, or hangman.

Supporting hobbies for men and women

Here are some past hobbies and corresponding activities for you to mull over and add your own ideas too.

The knitter
Provide old knitting patterns to look through and a rummage bag of different types of wool to feel. Make pom poms. Have some uncompleted knitted squares or ties that they may wish to help finish off.

"When it came to knitting I aways asked the ladies to help me cast on. One lady's dementia was too progressed for her to help me to do this but she was able to untangle a ball of wool and she sat there happily helping me for ages."

Jo Whitehouse, activity co-ordinator

The DIY enthusiast
Bring in an old tool box and tool belt or an apron to get down to work. Find things such as nuts and bolts for the older person

to sort through and match up, or ask them to tighten screws into pieces of wood or connect smaller PVC pipes together.

The car fanatic

If an older person's passion was cars, bring in pictures of old cars or smaller engine parts. Name different types of cars, bring in a toy car collection. Watch car racing DVDs and how to clean an engine or change a tyre films on YouTube. Maybe you could wash a car together.

The gardener

The lover of gardening might enjoy looking through gardening magazines or seed catalogues. Provide the older person with a place to plant seeds, water them and watch them grow. Harvest vegetables, create a herb garden. Being outdoors can be beneficial for people with dementia, you could encourage them to rake leaves, or press flowers in books and then make pictures with them.

The music lover

Try 'name that tune' or instrument quizzes. Bring in favourite pieces of music and instruments. Sing together, make music together, explore different rhythms and repeating call and response simple tunes on different instruments. Be a conductor for a day, provide a conductor baton to conduct along to favourite classical music.

The sports fan

Watch sporting highlights, from their favourite era perhaps, or access old footage on YouTube. Keep them active and provide the avid sports lover with the chance to mini put, do Wii bowling, and all the other sports games that are available. Encourage outdoor bowls, and softball cricket, and bring in sporting memorabilia to touch and discuss thereby stimulating memories. Play audio recordings from favourite games to stimulate imagination.

The travel lover
Download google earth to an iPad or tablet, ask what wonders and places they would like to see and take them on a virtual tour. Let them dive into oceans to explore shipwrecks, visit places where they went on honeymoon, or were stationed overseas.

The animal lover
Unconditional love from an animal can be so healing. Patting animals can lower agitation and reduce a feeling of isolation. Encourage contact with pets, brushing a dog's fur might be enjoyed although the carer needs to be mindful that hands must be washed well after contact. Feeding fish can engender a feeling of responsibility. An aquarium containing tropical fish could be a delight. Tortoises, hamsters, rabbits, budgies, cats can all bring comfort and connection. Watching funny animal extracts on YouTube together can be fun and a happy distraction. Bring in story books about animals. Play animal snap. Some people communicate more readily with a pet than humans, but ask the individual, as not everyone likes animals, there may be fear or indeed allergies.

"In the middle to late stages of Alzheimer's, some people are comforted by holding a stuffed kitten or puppy. Consider, when you are leaving an elder, providing them with an animatronic animal or battery operated one for comfort and companionship."

Terri, carer

"One of our residents used to have a horse I discovered. She had been very low and hadn't spoken for weeks so one day I asked management if I could bring my pony into the garden for her. The effect was incredible, she stroked her, talked to her, eyes sparkling, and many of the residents talked about this and enjoyed my pony too."

Kate, senior carer

The parent and homemaker
For people with dementia doing household chores can help them retain dignity and a sense of purpose. Therapeutic chores can include: folding sheets; washing up; polishing shoes; sweeping; filling bird feeders; preparing vegetables; or arranging flowers.

Interactions with children and babies have been a normal part of that person's life as a parent so create opportunities for interaction with children, arranging for children to sing or read to them, or taking a walk to a playground. People with dementia have a higher level of positive engagement when interacting with children and are able to teach children things, such as how to fold a towel, how to dust handrails or how to categorise things by seasons or colours. There are some risks and challenges to facilitating intergenerational activities so vigilant supervision could be necessary. Both children and people with dementia can be unpredictable and lack inhibitions, so caution must be taken to ensure the safety of both parties.

Dolls and soft toy therapy in dementia care

Alternative therapies such as doll therapy are becoming more common as an alternative to drug intervention. Some older adults, particularly women, may enjoy holding and caring for a baby doll. Often, the person connects with that baby doll and enjoys the sense of a familiar role in caregiving for it. Life like or reborn dolls can help comfort and reduce stress and agitation and allow for a flow of communication by triggering happy memories. Emotional expression may come with a feeling of responsibility and care for a baby. Sometimes they can help bring someone with dementia out of their shell, however if you or your care setting are wishing to use reborn dolls as therapy for people with dementia, it is important for staff to be able to feel confident explaining to the person's relatives why the therapy is beneficial. Sometimes relatives can be upset by seeing their loved ones in what they perceive as an infantilised state. It is important as a carer that you monitor an older person's interaction with the dolls carefully. Some care homes have found residents can get too attached to the dolls, putting them to sleep in their beds, for example, while they sleep in the chair.

Creativity and the arts in dementia care

Creativity allows access to emotions, thoughts, self-exploration, hopes and dreams. Being engaged in the arts provides wonderful opportunities for people with dementia to express themselves.

Do

- *Remember* that a person's ability to engage in an activity will change over the course of dementia, so it is important to regularly review which activities the person responds to.
- *Encourage* the person or group to be spontaneous, allowing for free joyful expression.

- *Give* as many opportunities as possible for interacting and relating to others where appropriate.
- *Provide* a consistent and heartfelt approach minimising distractions.
- *Focus* on abilities rather than problems.
- *Join* people where they are in time and place and consider the world from their perspective.

ART

An elder's still vibrant imagination is strengthened through therapeutic art. Art provides a creative outlet to make something, so it provides a purpose and a task. Gather some non-toxic clay, water colour paints, washable markers, coloured pens or pencils, and paper. You can use these materials in a directed way, "Today let's try to paint a rainbow" or a non-directed way, "Feel free to paint anything you feel like". Clay and paint are great for tactile stimulation and they provide a way to occupy and strengthen the hands as well. Other ideas that are failure free include:

- finger painting to music – put primary colours onto the fingers of each hand and "play the piano" to the tune and rhythm;
- doodling – with eyes closed let the felt tip pen move where it will;
- making charity cards – through stencilling or rubber stamping;
- fabric painting.

MUSIC

We can communicate through the power of music. Music may be able to connect us where words cannot. Music enriches the brain and nourishes the spirit. Listening and responding to music is a great stress reliever and can be a good source of pain management, provide distraction and improve sleep patterns. Those with dementia will show a greater freedom and spontaneity and may wish to move and dance to the music. People in the early to mid-stages of Alzheimer's may be able to sing in a choir or play the piano (see www.verywell.com). *Music for the brain* is a very good initiative. Through the process of participating in singing an elder may be able to access long or short term memories and enjoy reminiscing. If an elder enjoys listening to music rather than performing it, make recordings of favourite songs.

"A favourite song can bring back a thousand memories, maybe happy or sad but a part of the brain never forgets the songs, their lyrics or the meaning they had to us. In far too many cases to mention we have had residents in the late stages of dementia that rarely speak but will sing along to every word of a favourite song. Building a personal play list for each individual can be very helpful and can ease agitation and lift their mood if feeling down."

Jo Whitehouse, Head of Activities,
Sonnet Care Homes

Tips for involving music in activities

- Put on some of their old time dance favourites and dance.
- Listen to some recordings that hold meaning for that person (church music, hits from their youth, etc.). Play one at a time and discuss its meaning.

- Create a play list on an iPod for them.
- Try humming when assisting to dress (this can be calming).
- Write a list of the activities that get the best response.
- Play musical instruments together, tambourines, drums, recorders, bells.
- Try wireless headphones or personal audiotape, CD or MP3 players with headphones, as music that is invigorating to one person may cause agitation in another.

Don't

- Persist with certain pieces if the person you are caring for becomes agitated. Some music can just become noise. (Try again another day, if it happens again make a note of it for future reference.)
- Immediately turn off music that provokes a tearful response, ask if they are okay and if they are upset. Talk about why the music made them feel emotional. It could be a hymn that was played at a funeral or a song that touched them at the time they first heard it. These feelings are important for emotional health too. Embrace them and move on to something else when the piece has finished.

Caroline J Benham,
www.brightcopperkettles.co.uk

The power of the drum
I am often asked to go into care homes not only to train the staff, but to talk about the importance of care that honours and celebrates with the relatives and residents too. I use my drum, having been trained in native American traditions, to softly play like a heartbeat over each older person where the ritual of recognition of the life of that elder begins. I

state that the echoes of the drum honour and recognise the journey of their family and themselves till this point in time, celebrating all that they are, all that they have been, all that they will be. I love seeing the mixed response of tears, surprise, relief, peace and laughter, the soul healing that comes when someone truly takes the time to honour and celebrate the life of another.

I have led drum circles with elders for many years and I recommend you organise one, as the benefits are so positive and far reaching.

- It brings laughter and delight.
- It gives elders a voice and a way to communicate and release emotions, both negative and positive.
- They know that they can be heard and respond through the drum even if they have lost language skills.
- Drumming induces alpha brain waves which make elders feel calm and relaxed.
- It helps keep elders in the present moment.
- It is failure free.
- It is fun and socially inclusive and brings people together.

CONSIDER

Try and use different sounding drums and percussion instruments e.g. bongos, small djembes – middle sound, buffalo drums and djembes – bass, ocean drum and thunder tube – natural sounds, and shakers. We instinctively possess a sense of rhythm. We can tap our feet, our hearts beat, we use a rhythm to walk, we dance to a rhythm. We march to the beat of our own drum in life!

The power of poetry

Most people over sixty were taught to recite classic poems by heart at school and the reassurance that can be had from hearing familiar words can be most uplifting. For someone who is aware that they struggle to remember things, this sense of recall can be both reassuring and give a sense of achievement. We use the same part of the brain to remember poetry as to remember song lyrics. Read poetry aloud together, perhaps they can still recite Wordsworth from their school days.

The power of story telling

Together, you could introduce music, a story or poem or song to illustrate and celebrate some past memories of those in your care setting. Involving older people in this way restores the storytelling role to elders. Story telling sparks memories, encourages communication and promotes self-esteem among those with dementia. Familiar and favourite stories can be effectively used as well as personal memory stories. New spontaneous ones can be created together. Include props, mimes and taking different roles.

Tips for storytelling

- Remember this is an opportunity for an elder to create their own narrative, to have control in some ways over what happens. To re-create their own story can restore self-esteem and communication.
- There is no wrong or right way, storytelling is failure free and can be as expansive or minimalist as the participants' imagination will allow them to be. So throw out rules, storytelling in this context does not require

a beginning, middle, or end. Be free in creative story-telling, a flow of nonsensical characters or ideas can be liberating, thrilling and laughter inducing too.

- Remember you can tell a story without words, using grunts, sounds, music, even gobbledygook.
- For inspiration you could use two objects to be woven into the story or a visual aid such as a picture. Enjoy choosing pictures that can stimulate the imagination, family photos are not so successful as they can limit imagination, often the more unrealistic the picture, the better. Large, colourful pictures for example of animals dressed as humans, or unusual settings and scenarios like a spaceman in a supermarket, can work really well.
- You will find more engagement if you use open-ended questions such as, "What should we call the person?", "Where are they going?", "What sounds do you hear in the picture?", "What could this be?", "What is going on here?" Involve music by asking, "What might she be singing?" or "What music does the character like?"
- Accept any participation, be it just unintelligible noises, repeat back to enable a feeling of validation and incorporation.
- All ideas are valid and a spring board for creative opportunity.
- Set aside judgements or the need to control and enjoy the ride!

"People with dementia can express themselves quite beautifully through imagination in creative storytelling. Removing the pressure to remember had such a profound impact on the seniors' level of engagement that it changed how their communities saw them. They were no longer invisible, but were now 'storytellers'."

Anne Basting, Timeslips

Reminiscence

Encourage relatives to bring in photographs showing important places, and people. Reminiscence work can be beneficial
to create links between the past and the present and enable a
person to develop a sense of self-worth and individual identity.
Ideas for themes can include childhood, school days, family
life, an evening out, the queen's coronation, adjusting to life
after the war, rationing, first loves, and favourite holidays.

"I ask people to think back to when they used to get ready for
a special evening out. I ask them to describe what they did,
from washing their hair to putting on make-up or Brylcreem
and we act it out."

Sally, carer

Ideas for later stages of dementia

Remember to involve all the senses where possible.

Do

- Stimulate daily experiences from the past, for example
  placing feet in water or sand to trigger reminiscences and
  shared memories.
- Use twiddle muffs, which are knitted woollen muffs
  with items such as ribbons, large buttons or textured
  fabrics attached to them. Patients with dementia can
  twiddle them in their hands. People with dementia
  often have restless hands and like something to keep
  them occupied. The warm cosiness of the muff also has
  a calming effect. Go online to find patterns and instructions for how to make them.

You could also try

- vibrating or moving sensations, massage or touched based therapies, rocking, stroking, hand massage;
- water based activities;
- sensory blankets, cushions, aprons;
- objects with tactile qualities of rough/smooth, hot/cold, or beads and buttons;
- looking for objects in a bowl of rice or lentils;
- rummaging boxes with a range of interesting objects, fabrics or things of particular personal significance;
- treasure chests containing surprising, unexpected things;
- dressing up items such as gloves, hats, scarves;
- coloured paper and wool for tearing, folding, winding and making collages;
- memory boxes and memorabilia from the past, old games, tools, pictures;
- dolls and soft toys;
- stacking cups;
- blowing bubbles;
- singing;
- nature boxes, moss, pinecones, bark, flower petals, seeds, pictures of birds, recordings of nature;
- sound effects and sound quizzes;
- smelling herbs, scented plants, washing soaps from the past;
- a different selection of tastes from the past, sweets, jams etc.

Making sensory mats

Use sensory mats to provide a soothing and stimulating activity. The size of your fidget mat is up to you. It can be positioned on a table with velcro.

Take a piece of strong, brightly coloured cotton material, place mat size or larger. Use your imagination; anything interesting and safe that is suitable. Decorations should be securely attached to fabric for safety reasons.

For example: Sew on a zipper, attach buttons, make a button hole for large buttons with button flaps, sew in a bunch of wool strands (about 7 inches/18cm – to be braided). Attach belt and buckle, sew in a fluffy piece of fabric and leather, attach pom-poms, squish toys, and more. Attach soft toys, sew in a little pocket, large colourful beads, key ring etc.

Tips

Mats may be personalised, e.g. if the older person was a hairdresser, attach things she would recognise and enjoy to touch.

You may wish to make it into an apron by placing ribbons on the sides.

CONSIDER

If an individual is bed bound, create an activity plan that will bring both pleasure, comfort and stimulation and enable the elder to have things to look at, touch, smell or listen to. Bring the outside world into the world of an elder. You are world makers when their world has shrunk to three feet around their bed, so see this as a rewarding opportunity to make a difference. Have a box containing materials and objects of different textures, velvet, hessian, an orange, silk hanky, beads. Encourage each individual to touch the items, and see if by touch alone they can guess what they are. Give the older person an opportunity to smell different perfumes or aftershaves. See if they can remember a favourite scent they used to wear.

"I have always believed that having dementia should not stop anyone from being able to continue doing the things they have always enjoyed. Although we have a duty of care to make sure the residents are safe 'wrapping them in cotton wool' is not always the answer. I am forever searching for new things we can do together. Last year I went for a short break in a caravan to Mersea Island. While I was there I kept thinking of how some of our residents would enjoy this. So six months later (and after quite a bit of planning) we took four of our residents there for the weekend. The normality of it and the smell of the sea air had such a wonderful effect."

Jo Whitehouse, Head of Activities,
Sonnet Care Homes

7

How to Care as Relatives
for Loved Ones

"The pain now is part of the happiness then."

C S Lewis

This chapter is especially for you who are caring at home for a member of the family, to hold your hand, to be a friend, to provide emotional and practical support with extra hints and tips to assist your caring role, whether your loved one has dementia or they are being cared for by you at the end of their lives.

I cared for both my parents till the end of their lives. I moved from London to West Sussex to be near them. I tried to give them the support that they needed but it was not always smooth sailing! I was a single mother and, having moved from London, did not have a support network of friends and family, so I understand the emotional rollercoaster, physical exhaustion, and deep aloneness that can be overwhelming at times when you are caring for elder loved ones.

My time with them was full of moments of love, frustration, laughter, despair, grief and healing. I learnt so much during that time – about them, myself, my limitations, my resilience, my fears and my capacity for love.

As our parents become older, more frail and less able we may see this as an opportunity to care for them at the end stages of their lives, with love and gratitude for the care and support they gave us at the beginning of our own. However this reversal of child and parent roles can be difficult and unsettling.

"It is difficult for me to relate to this vulnerable and frail person, where is the capable and caring mother I once knew? I know it must be especially confusing and at times frightening for her, but I miss my Mum"

Anna, carer

Looking after elder relatives and loved ones can prove satisfying but also challenging as it will generally follow a sudden change, crisis, or deterioration in their health. You may also be struggling with caring for your own family and pursuing a career. Perhaps your relationship with your elder relatives is strained and fraught and this too can require delicate navigation so that resentments and bitterness do not build up.

"Can we still have a relationship or only that of carer/patient?"

Dee, carer

Caring for yourself

However much care we give our elderly loved ones, a decline in health and strength, despite our best efforts, is so painful to watch. When caring for a loved one our life revolves around that person, our world can shrink and it can feel like an overwhelming or impossible task. Add to this the complicated family dynamics as well as your own fear of losing someone that you love, either to dementia, a care home, or through death, and stress levels can become very high. Fifty-two per cent of carers have been treated for stress because of their caring role. So it is important that you find good coping mechanisms and strategies to help yourself.

Please read the How to Care for Yourself and Prevent Burnout section but also consider the following tips.

- Consult other family members to share responsibility. Co-ordinate times when family or friends could care for your loved one to give you a weekend break to rest and recharge.
- Delegate. Find ways to outsource some tasks to lighten your load.
- Consider using daycare to give you a break in the day. Could someone do your ironing or housework? Perhaps you could think about using meals on wheels.
- Join a support group. Spending time with others who understand can alleviate some of the loneliness and provide positive sharing of suggestions.
- Try meditation or yoga, there are lots of mobile phone apps that you can follow if you can't get out of the house. Headspace is a good meditation app.
- Keep physically active as it will strengthen your immune system and increase your production of endorphins and this will make you feel better.
- Build some **you** time into your day. Have a massage, go for a swim or a walk, visit a church, have tea with a friend.
- Try to bear in mind your family and personal values

when caring for a relative, our values are what we draw on to cope with the ups and downs of family life and can play an important part in how we care for them in later life.

Below are the details of some organisations you could approach for help and to lighten your load.

Women's Royal Voluntary Service
Find out where your nearest local one is. They offer a choice of services, including visiting schemes, home delivered meals, and volunteer drivers.
www.royalvoluntaryservice.org.uk
www.wrvs.org.uk

Revitalise
It offers special Alzheimer's holidays for people with dementia and their carers, which are subsidised by the Alzheimer's Society.
www.revitalise.org.uk
Tel 08453 451 970

Crossroads Care
This is Britain's leading provider of support for carers and the people they care for. www.crossroadscare.org.uk
Tel 08454 500 350

Age UK
Provides information, support and grants for all aspects of elder care and support for those looking after someone with dementia.
www.ageuk.org.uk
Advice line 08001 696 565

Alzheimer's Society

It has information about caring for someone with dementia and offers an online forum. www.alzheimers.org.uk

Emotional crisis

It is quite normal to feel lonely, misunderstood, unappreciated and angry about what is happening to the people we love. Sometimes it becomes necessary to make unpopular decisions about "what is best" for our loved ones and this can make us feel as if we are letting them down or even betraying them, which means decisions get delayed until a crisis forces our hand.

"The emotional fall out of anger, frustration, fear and anxiety overwhelms me"

Trish, carer

"Guilt comes with the territory, always I felt I should be somewhere else, everyone got short shrift. Let alone taking time for myself."

Elizabeth, carer

Guilt is a common emotion when caring for an elderly relative. How do you juggle your other responsibilities, like work and children, while caring for your elder parent? Feeling torn between the demands of adult children, grandchildren, our career and ageing parents can result in feeling overwhelmed, resentful, and ashamed at not coping. All kinds of complex reactions to problems and difficult relationships within families can get triggered at these times. The situation can be even worse if you live a long way from your parents and you want to do your best for them but you also need to live your own life.

"I am worried. Can I cope? Where is the person I love in all this?"

Toby, carer

"It feels like he's leaving me and there is nothing I can do about it."

Hannah, carer

This emotional turmoil can lead to stress, anxiety and depression. Do not suffer alone, reach out to friends, support groups, your GP and helpful organisations like the ones below.

Depression Alliance
Now merged with MIND, it helps people suffering from depression, offering information and advice as well as a network of support groups.
www.depressionalliance.org
Tel 08451 232 320
www.mind.org.uk

National Association for Mental Health (MIND)
Offers support to people in mental distress and their families.
www.mind.org.uk
Free advice line 02085 192 122

Sane
A mental health charity that supports those with anxiety or depression.
Tel 08457678000

Carers Trust
This is a comprehensive site providing information, advice and support services to carers.

www.carers.org
Tel 08448 004 361

Elderly Parents
Provides information for adult children caring for elderly parents.
www.elderlyparents.org.uk

Carers UK
Their website offers a comprehensive range of information for carers.
www.carersuk.org
Free carers line 0808 808 777

Keeping your loved one safe

Be aware of abuse. A UK study found that 342,400 people aged over sixty-six years living in private households reported mistreatment by a family member, close friend, caseworker or neighbour. If you suspect your relative has been abused it is important that you talk to them about it. If they choose to take the matter forward you need to report any incident to the safeguarding team at social services. These teams take responsibility for investigating allegations of abuse in response to "safeguarding alerts". If your relative lacks mental capacity to make the decision about whether to report suspected abuse to social services you can do it for them by "acting in their best interest".

Action on Elder Abuse
Works to protect and prevent the abuse of vulnerable older people.
www.elderabuse.org.uk
Free helpline 0808 808 8141

Dignity
For support and online forum
dignityincare.org.uk

Caring for a loved one with dementia

Dementia is one of the main causes of disability in later life, ahead of some cancers, cardiovascular disease and stroke. It is important to recognise that you will need to treat yourself gently because it can be so painful to watch someone you know and love change, possibly quite dramatically, into someone you no longer know. You may feel bereaved as you have to come to terms with the knowledge that you may have "lost" the person you knew. Part of the sense of bereavement may stem from losing the person you have always turned to for advice and support as your relationship changes and you begin to feel like the "parent" while the parent becomes as vulnerable as your child.

But remember it is never too late to tell someone that you love them and find ways to honour the life you shared as you adjust to a new way of being together.

"You will need to travel light, and learn how to be flexible, to find new routes to familiar places, to throw away all of the old maps, all of the old guides. You are on a trip that will demand all of your patience, your stamina, and your love."
Tom and Karen Brenner, Alzheimers reading room

As your loved one faces losses of memory and senses allow yourself space to grieve for the losses you are enduring, tend to yourself, seek help.

TAKING POSITIVE STEPS

Caring for a loved one with dementia involves ensuring that they keep active and engaged as much as possible. This can sometimes be difficult to maintain, so it is essential that you take steps to make things easier for everyone involved.

Caroline J Benham, Bright Copper Kettles, contributes these tips.

Do

- try to talk positively to your loved one about dementia;
- attend a Dementia Friends session;
- encourage your loved one to think about supporting a dementia charity or perhaps hold a coffee morning at your home with friends and family;
- arrange for Dementia Friends sessions to be given at any clubs that they attend;
- attend your local Dementia Cafe, Music for the Brain or similar groups;
- contact the Alzheimer's Society to ask about their "Befriending Service";
- speak to friends about the diagnosis – you may find that you are the one that needs support the most;
- try to continue with ongoing interests (watching or playing sports, lunches with friends, walking groups, knitting groups, etc.).

Don't

- try to force the person you are caring for to accept the diagnosis, it can sometimes just be a matter of time;
- pressure them to go out with friends, especially if you know they are tired.

Note: Large groups can be daunting for someone with dementia although it will often depend on the activity. A barn dance or singing group can be great fun – everyone is trying to "have a go" so your loved one will often just feel part of the group. A large dinner party where everyone is talking at once can prove too much and it may be best to avoid these types of events if this becomes apparent. If you notice that the person you care for avoids going out without you (even with friends), it may be because they are becoming afraid of not being able to cope without you.

The Dementia Assistance Card has been designed to help those with dementia or memory loss who might get into difficulties in public places. The cards share information about names and contact numbers of relatives, friends or care homes in the event of emergency. Having one may serve to reassure. Visit dementiaassistancecard.com for further information.

Keep it simple

On days that you have appointments or family celebrations to attend keep "everyday" activities as simple as possible. This will keep distractions to a minimum to help them focus on what is important.

Do

- prepare the breakfast table the night before;
- keep choices to a minimum, serve a favourite dish at mealtimes;
- keep conversations simple with low key subjects;
- discuss outfits earlier in the week if it matters what your loved one wears for the occasion, lay it out ready on the day and try to have an alternative to hand too;
- allow time for pain relief, if required, to work before attempting anything physical (remember this can mean getting out of bed for some people).

Don't

- hurry;
- offer too many choices (ever!), keep to two or three max;
- get upset or annoyed if your loved one sits down to breakfast in the outfit they intend to wear for the party that evening (that's why you sorted a spare!).

Mealtimes for your loved one

Having dementia can sometimes cause confusion around meal times and someone suffering from dementia may not recognise when they are hungry or thirsty, or what types of foods are suitable to eat together. Lemon curd and pickle sandwiches may be easy to prepare but wouldn't necessarily be their usual choice!

Do

- offer food and drinks at regular intervals;
- keep portions small (a full plate can put someone off entirely if they don't feel hungry);
- try a linked activity before a meal to promote hunger (a fishing game before Fisherman's Pie, topping a pizza before it is cooked);
- try offering a couple of chocolates or a sweet biscuit before a meal;
- where appropriate, buy non-alcoholic alternatives if medication means no alcohol;
- use food and drink as an activity, bake a cake or a loaf of bread to enjoy with morning coffee;
- encourage food preparation for meals, prepare vegetables together, mix sauces, etc.

Don't

- deny foods or drinks even if they've just eaten, offer small snacks instead (try saying, "it's not ready yet, would you like a piece of cheese while we're waiting?");
- give them too much to do for a single task (e.g. prepare the carrots together, if they are only able to do one or two they won't notice that you have done the majority and will have a feeling of accomplishment when they see everything is prepared).

Helping each other

Some people find that their emotional needs are not met when they have dementia. It can be hard to feel needed when you are being cared for. Try to find different ways to help to fill this gap with something that suits the person you are caring for.

Do

- encourage feeding any pets you have, keep a chart next to the food to note when they have been fed;
- use a specially designed dementia clock which shows day and time of day to help with self organising;
- offer to look after a pet when the owner is away;
- offer to walk a neighbour's dog;
- ask friends and family to bring their pets when visiting.

Reminiscence

Our personal histories are important to us, they help give focus to our thoughts and help others to connect with us. It is helpful, therefore, to create items that will assist with recalling the past and the people who are closest to your loved one.

Do

- Organise a photo album which depicts close family and friends (use a range of between one and three pictures per page).
- Use an online resource to create a printed version of your photo album, which includes a caption below each photo to name the person(s) in the picture ("my brother, Jack").
- If you enjoy creating the online album, consider creating others to include copies of favourite drawings by children or grandchildren, or favourite places, etc.

- Write a contents list to match your iPod play list. Include notes of why each track was chosen.
- Write out a family tree. This can be a useful prompt for names for your loved one, as well as a tool for conversation for other carers.
- Create a Memory Box for important dates. Memory Boxes are small, themed collections which can include a few photographs and other memorabilia referring to things that were significant in the elder's life. Wedding memories could be treasured through a garter, veil or other item worn on the day, a wedding certificate (or photocopy), photographs, rice or confetti. Memories of children could be stimulated or retained by looking at photographs, drawings, cards, birth certificates, a favourite toy that has been preserved, a hospital band, teeth, a hair curl, a nappy, or even Johnson's baby powder and lotion. If the person's employment or career was very important to them the box could contain a payslip and other items pertinent to their job. For example if they worked in an office these could be stationery, pens, paperclips or if they worked in a shoe factory, strips of leather, laces, Blakey's SEGS, small hammer.

Planning outings

When you care for someone with dementia, it's easy to become isolated out of fear that social situations will be stressful. This does not have to be the case! With some planning and thought an outing can be a very rewarding and welcome change of pace to the daily routine. To prepare . . .

Do

- Check distance and assess what will be tolerable for your loved one. Allow extra time.
- Plan the outing around the time of day they seem to have most energy.
- Consider the setting. Do they enjoy children being present or not?
- Prepare others for the special needs of your loved ones, call ahead to the restaurant or speak discreetly with the waiter before you are seated. Share information on a card that could say things like whether you will be ordering for them, how best to address your loved one and any special seating needs and dietary requirements.
- Remain calm and anticipate an enjoyable event. If you are nervous about things going well, that anxiety will be projected onto the person with dementia who can be strongly affected by the emotions of people around them.

With thanks to contributor Caroline J Benham, www.bright-copperkettles.co.uk

Please ensure you read the section on How to Care for Someone with Dementia and the dementia sections in all the other chapters too.

Caring for a loved one at end of life

Many people prefer to die at home, surrounded by familiar belongings and where loved ones can come and go. If you and your dying relative want this option then talk though the practicalities with your GP, district nurse or Macmillan nurse. They will be your main source of support and will help you arrange the supply of specialist equipment, such as an air mattress or lifting equipment, with the local health authority.

Although rewarding, caring for someone at home can be physically and emotionally demanding. You need to think about your own needs, have breaks to sleep and re-charge and find extra help to give you the support you will need.

"Some family members can do some things and others can't. Talk. Tell your family/friends what you feel able to do and certainly what you can't. But my experience is that it will always fall more heavily on someone's shoulders. And how does this get dealt with without unneeded fireworks? Talk. Take time away from the patient to talk to each other. Accept help. Friends don't have the emotional hook you may have but sometimes that helps us see the wood for the trees."

Elizabeth Purcell MSc,
CEO The Lewis Manning Trust

Be prepared for this to be an intense time which needs patience and understanding as well as a willingness to communicate openly and truthfully with the rest of the family.

- You may feel resentful if the rest of the family are not helping, sibling rivalry can surface and divide loyalties, too.
- You may find it impossible to think of anything else apart from preparing for your loved one's death.
- You may feel as if you are in a bubble, unable to relate to "normal life" as everyday conversations seem trivial and irrelevant in comparison.
- You may find restaurants and supermarkets too hard to handle, too loud, noisy, intrusive.
- You may feel the responsibility is overwhelming.

- You may entertain thoughts like, "I wish this was over!" and feel guilty for thinking them. Does this mean you do not love that person? Of course not. Does it make you a poor or heartless caregiver? No! It means you are human. You share these unspoken feelings with many other caregivers.

Do

- Give your suffering a voice and tell someone you trust, someone who can understand and not judge you.
- Tell friends what is happening and ask for practical help with laundry perhaps, or stocking up your fridge and freezer with homemade meals, soups etc.
- Explain what you are going through to your children and other family members.
- Employ a night nurse to stay over so you can have a night of uninterrupted sleep.
- Offer friends and family the opportunity to sit with your loved one.
- Attend a caregiver support group.
- Let off steam by exercising, journaling, painting or even breaking something you will not miss!

Please ensure you read the sections on How to Give Compassionate End of Life Care and How to Support Spiritual and Emotional Needs.

Addressing end of life decisions

Many of us are concerned about the end of our loved one's life and how we can support them to die with dignity in a place of their choosing. I often say a good life needs a good ending.

Doing this involves helping our relatives to plan ahead and look into the options that may or may not be possible. This means having a conversation with our loved one to find out what their preferences are before they are too poorly to communicate or unable to make their own decisions. It is a sensitive time but you will feel greatly relieved when you are sure that you know what your loved ones wishes are so that you will able to put them in place to the best of your ability.

End of life treatment decisions are made in the context of deeply held beliefs and personal opinions about what contributes to or constitutes your loved one's quality of life. Two questions that may help someone close to the end of life think about this are:

- what makes your life worth living now?; and
- what would make your life not worth living in the future?

You may discover that your relative wishes to ensure that the small things they value in everyday life continue if they become incapacitated. They may want to consider making a **living will**. This is a statement expressing a person's views on how they would like to be treated if in the future they are unable to make decisions for themselves. In order to be legally binding the living will must meet certain requirements at the time it is signed. It must be clear that the individual making the will:

- has the mental capacity to make the medical decisions contained in the living will;
- understands the consequences of these decisions;
- makes clear their wishes regarding future treatment; and
- makes the decision voluntarily and not under anyone else's influence.

Pro-choice living will offers a living will that has been put together by leading lawyers, doctors and nurses. If your relative has made a living will you should ensure you review what they have expressed periodically to ensure their wishes have not changed.

www.livingwill.org.uk

Tel 08707 777 868

Your relative may also want to consider an **advance directive**, a decision to refuse treatment, or an **advance statement**, any other decision about how the individual wishes to be treated. For example if the only treatment for your relative is aggressive chemotherapy or radical surgery, they may wish to opt for palliative care, which is about relieving symptoms and especially supplying effective pain relief. These directives and statements may be in the form of a signed and witnessed document/card or oral statement, or as a discussion note recorded in their medical file at your relative's request. It may give instructions regarding medical treatment and the request or refusal for life sustaining treatment. Your loved one may decide to place a Do Not Attempt Resuscitation (**DNAR**) in their medical notes.

Can you find out if they wish to donate their organs upon their death?

Funeral wishes

"I felt so much better knowing that mum and I had discussed her funeral plans, because in the midst of my grief at losing her I knew she was getting the send-off she wanted without me worrying if I had done it right for her."

Jane

Do not feel you need to get answers all at once to what their wishes may be, just make notes as and when appropriate opportunities allow for this kind of conversation. The following are questions you can sensitively ask your loved one to help you arrange what they would like.

- Would you like to be buried or cremated? (The majority of people choose to be cremated but if your loved one wishes to be buried you must purchase a plot with your funeral plan beforehand.)
- What sort of coffin would you prefer? (Choices might be wicker, or wooden, or to have a shroud.)
- Would you like flowers, and if so would you like to choose them?
- Would you like donations to a charity or charities of your choice, and if so which?
- Where would you like your service to be held?
- What music would you like and when?
- What hymns or readings would you like?
- Who would you like to speak at your funeral?
- Who would you like to conduct the funeral?
- Are there personal words you would like to write to be read out at your funeral?
- Would you like there to be a wake afterwards and if so where would you like the wake to be held?
- Do you have any requests for food or drink for the wake, or music?

The Natural Death Centre
provides information about woodland burials, cardboard coffins, living wills, funeral wishes forms and do it yourself funerals.
www.naturaldeath.org.uk
Tel 01962 712 690

Age UK
provide information about all aspects of end of life planning
and care as well as what to do when someone dies.
www.ageuk.org.uk

Funeral celebrants
If you wish to find details of possible celebrants you could try
www.funeralcelebrants.org.uk

Amanda Waring as a celebrant
If you want to contact me in this capacity go to
amandawaringevents.com
amandakwaring@icloud.com

Living funerals and celebrations of life

Amongst my other roles I am also a celebrant. In the past thirty
years I have led hundreds of ceremonies that are heart filled
and personalised, helping those who require my services to
celebrate life events in a memorable way.

I often conduct **celebration of life ceremonies** which can
take place even before death. These are also known as **living
funerals** and can enable you to honour your loved one's final
rite of passage, and say goodbye to each other in community,
surrounded by loved ones. Preparing for death as a rite of
passage can be creative, instructive, and full of life affirming
activities. I have been blessed with many spiritual teachers in
my life, and draw from many cultures and traditions when
creating bespoke ceremonies for those who ask me.

One ceremony that I take with families is an *aya despacho*,
it is a beautiful ritual to lovingly assist our cherished ones to
die consciously. It is a ceremony that has been practised for
hundreds of years in the Andes of South America and provides

deep celebration for the life of the individual who is in the process of departing. This ritual brings loving closure and an understanding of death, allowing and honouring that which must die.

An *aya despacho* is a prayer bundle prepared in gratitude to the earth, the mountains and the spirits that support us in this world. It can be a simple offering with few ingredients or it can be an elaborate affair. During a traditional *despacho* ceremony, participants build the *despacho* together by assembling various ingredients (each representing a symbolic element) and adding their own individual prayers of gratitude for that person and their life. An *aya despacho* allows participants to build a rainbow bridge for their loved one to the next world. Children and grandchildren can be involved in this heartfelt but joyous ceremony as you give thanks and deep gratitude for the life of that loved one, and they can take in the love and honouring whilst still physically with us.

These prayer bundles are traditionally either buried or offered to a sacred fire after the ceremony is completed.

With a knapsack on his back, a bindle

I will share an example of a simple ceremony, inspired by the *despacho* ceremony, which I have created with young grandchildren. They can do it with you at the bedside of their grandparent.

To create the knapsack/bindle
Get a metre square cloth of any bright colour you choose. Open it out and say that you are making a special knapsack/bindle for the grandparent to take with them on their next journey. You will fill it with your wishes, prayers and gifts.

Into this cloth you can place any small things the children

feel drawn to give, and the reason for them should be shared. Each gift that goes into the centre of the cloth, can be blown onto with a breath of love if you choose. Examples of items that could be included and the ideas that might go with them are:

- confetti stars – connection to the stars;
- colourful candy or sprinkles – to celebrate what their life meant to you;
- flower petals – for healing any regrets or sadness with compassion;
- corn – a gift back to the earth for what you have been given;
- raisins and dried fruits – for all the relatives that have passed over already;
- one chocolate coin – to ensure success;
- an image of a dove – to carry your prayers;
- rice – to bring prayers into fruition;
- sage or rosemary – for protection;
- chocolates – for all the kindness that person has given you;
- copies of photos of happy times, weddings, holidays;
- small drawings of rainbows, angels, smiling faces;
- small drawings of animals and loved companions;
- small drawing of water or the sea acknowledging the emotions and tears of those left behind;
- love hearts – honouring the love that is shared.

Once the knapsack/bindle material is full of goodies and wishes the corners of the cloth can be brought together and you can tie this onto a bamboo stick. There is the knapsack/bindle, a bit like Dick Whittington's, ready for the grandparent's next journey. This can stay in the elder's room providing something tangible, heartfelt and comforting for that elder.

It can then be buried with the deceased or placed in the coffin for the cremation if wished.

Out of the mouths of babes

Children's involvement and indeed their point of view on death can be beautifully healing for the person departing and those left behind. When my father died and I told my son and his cousins, who were six and five at the time, they innocently but joyfully raced to the trampoline, jumped up and down and chanted, "Hooray grandpa's gone to heaven, hooray he is in heaven". My son could see my tears and asked, "Mummy if heaven's such a nice place, why are people so sad about going there?" "Heaven's like a nice hotel," he continued, "and the first thing the angels will say to Grandpa is 'this way to the bar'!" I couldn't help laughing through my tears.

A personal service

When taking a funeral/ceremony my wish is to make the service a beautiful, uplifting, and healing experience for all who attend. In the midst of their grief, people won't always remember exactly what you said, but they will remember exactly how you made them feel. I feel very privileged to help families create the perfect ceremony or celebration, be it a religious service, multi faith or non-spiritual ceremony for their loved one. It is always an honour to get to know the life of that elder or person who has passed and write a memorable eulogy bringing comfort to those left behind.

I have conducted ceremonies in woods, castles, beaches,

gardens, and stone circles as well as in churches, synagogues and crematoriums. So when you are thinking about funeral planning do not forget that there are many options available for you.

Remembering our loved ones well is not only a tribute to the deceased; it strengthens our bonds as family and community. End-of-life ceremonies should uplift and connect us at a time when we may feel profound grief and disconnection, becoming celebrations of life lived.

Addressing regrets

The dying process of a close relative is a critical time for families and it can bring about a togetherness within an extended family unit which, though sad, can be a wonderful shared experience too. However the death, especially of the second parent, can bring back into focus family feuds and other unresolved issues which may have lain dormant for years. Think about how you might feel later once your loved one passes. Will there be words unsaid, hurts that have not healed and resentments still harboured? Could there be anything that you will regret later?

If there are any unresolved issues with your loved one and you feel it is too late to find the resolution or forgiveness you need, consider the Hawaiian *Ho' oponopono* mantra below. Saying this several times to your loved one even though they cannot answer may bring you some peace and acceptance.

> *I Love you*
> *I am sorry I . . .*
> *Please forgive me for . . .*
> *Thank you*
> *I love you*

Remember that people in a coma can sense and hear sounds around them so continue to talk to and touch them.

When my father was dying I was riddled with unexpressed rage at certain aspects of his behaviour that I had endured for so long without challenging him. I loved him fiercely but was frightened of him, particularly of his drunken rages, and rarely found the courage to stand up to him, choosing the path of acquiescence for fear of the consequences. I had to find some sort of resolution and forgiveness for him and myself, to allow for a "clean death" where we could both be liberated in our ultimate separation. To do this I knew I had to speak **my truth** to him. On the day of this unburdening, this releasing, truth telling, I felt calm and held Dad's hands as I spoke to him gently but freely about all aspects of our relationship. I asked if he would listen until I finished speaking, that it was important. I spoke for over an hour as the memories flowed through me. I asked for his forgiveness, as in the moment of speaking so honestly with him I could feel my forgiveness of him too. I thanked him for creating me and I thanked him for the challenges he gave me. I told him that his life had enriched me, that I had felt his love and that I would miss him, but now without my rage or anger I could let him go. I washed my father's feet and combed his hair and honoured him in a way that felt right for me. It was a profound life-changing experience and I could feel the peace and healing between us and so could he. That's why I share this memory, already described in *Heart of Care*, again.

The power of love

Although your loved one may not recall who you are, on a deeper level in that moment they will know how you made them feel. So, take time to sit and hold your loved one's hand, gently brush their hair, give a hand massage, a kiss, a hug.

They might not be able to demonstrate their appreciation, but will feel that comfort from your tender care. Expressing your love without expecting anything in return is a blessing and a true gift to be shared.

"I'd just like to say to my family that I love you all but there may be days to come when I can't."

Dave, dementia patient

Saying goodbye

Death is such a personal experience for the dying and they will go through this process regardless of our actions, which is why one can feel so helpless. Both your loved one and yourself may go through certain stages of grief; denial, anger, depression, bargaining. You may make a deal with God or a higher power in an attempt to stop the death, to not have to say goodbye, to prevent your feelings of helplessness. You may find that your loved one accepts that it is "their time" to go more readily than you do, they may be surrendering, when what you want is for them to fight and stay. This inner turmoil can eat one up inside. If your loved one is at peace with their situation try and find that place in your heart where you can let them go, gently and lovingly to ease their smooth transition.

Even if your loved one is unresponsive tell them how much you love them and talk with them about the happy memories you will have to treasure when they are gone. You can tell them that it is alright for them to go. Some people need "permission" to die and not be "tied" to life. If your faith dictates this you can reaffirm "you will see them again" and that you will hold onto the love and not the loss.

You may feel like saying words at the bedside in the form of a prayer or affirmation that can help the process of letting

go for both of you. You could see if something like this res-
onates with you.

"My heart is so full, I am acknowledging the love we share and
give thanks for all those cherished memories and experiences.
I release you now with love and peace knowing that our love
will never cease but flow across the summer lands, allowing
you to gently go to where your soul is calling you, to be free."

Amanda Waring

The dying moments

I sat with my beloved Granny when she was dying. She could no
longer speak and she was taking rasping, snoring, loud breaths
through an open mouth. Listening to it was uncomfortable.
I knew it was making her mouth dry so I wiped her lips and
mouth with a damp cloth. I wanted to feel peaceful with her, but
the noise of her breathing set me on edge. I felt guilty. I wanted
to feel more present with her but had to keep leaving the room.
I found it so upsetting and disconcerting. When Mum arrived
to share this time, Granny's breathing had changed again. It
alternated between the loud rasping breaths and quiet shallow
breathing. Then her breathing stopped ... and then it started
again ... and then it stopped and Mum and I looked at each other
tearfully thinking this was the moment of death ... and then
she started breathing again. Each time her breath stopped, Mum
and I seemed to hold our breath too, each moment felt heart
stopping for us, just not her. Granny seemed to stop breathing
for an eternity and then she would take another intake of breath.
This carried on for so long, Mum and I in a constant anticipation
of it being her final moment until ... until ... that we both got
the giggles, we couldn't stop ourselves. We were apologising to
Granny, tears streaming down our face with laughter and grief

all at once. I had never imagined that we would be laughing at the death bed but somehow it dissolved our tension. I hope Granny, a woman with a wonderful sense of fun, hearing the sounds of laughter and not tears, would have forgiven us.

What I did not know then was that this particular form of breathing is common. It is known as Cheyne-Stokes breathing and is part of the final dying process.

Since the death of my granny I have become a death doula or soul midwife, sitting with the dying and easing their passing where I can, and so I share this knowledge and my experience with you to help you where possible.

The final breath

It is not unusual for someone to hang on to life until a relative or friend arrives at their bedside, or until a special anniversary or birthday.

In contrast some people seem to make a deliberate choice to die alone. This can be heartbreaking if you only went on a short break and you may feel guilty that you let them down by missing that crucial moment, or hurt that they chose not to be with you at the moment of death. Be aware though that often it is easier for a dying person to let go when they are not tied to the presence of another

When death itself happens it can happen very quickly, sometimes the person will give several outward pants as their hearts and lungs stop. At the point of death people can often look years younger, as if all the cares and worries have gone. They can look remarkably peaceful. The moment of death can be experienced in many ways, it can feel an intensely spiritual moment or an anti-climax. You may feel grief, or relief, or numb. You may sense that the essence of the person has gone leaving the body just as an empty shell.

You may find being alone with the body both reassuring and sometimes unexpectedly peaceful. Some people have reported seeing something like a mist hovering over the body and then leaving. Other reports have described loving light filling the room, a beautiful perfume, or a sudden change in room temperature. Some have sensed a heaviness in the air, which seems to take some time to clear.

Friends and relatives who were not there have experienced "seeing" or "sensing" the loved one who has died and instinctively knowing the time of death. Such visitations bring comfort and assurance to many. "There are more things in heaven and earth . . ."

Contact any of the following organisations to give advice and help you support a dying relative.

Hospice Information Service
www.hospiceinformation.info

The Transitus Network
A network of people involved in supporting those that are dying in a sacred way
www.transitus.co.uk

Macmillan Cancer Line
Information on cancer and Macmillan nurses
www.macmillan.org.uk
Tel 0808 808 0000

Marie Curie Cancer Care
For information on cancer care and Marie Curie nurses
www.mariecurie.org.uk
Tel 0800716 146

Dying Matters
Information on what to expect during end of life care and
ideas for funerals and support
www.dyingmatters.org

Age UK
Information about all aspects of end of life planning and care
as well as what to do when someone dies
www.ageuk.org.uk

Final Fling
An informative website looking at death and dying
www.finalfling.com

Death Cafés
At death cafés people get together in a relaxed setting to safely
and informally discuss death along with cake and tea.
www.deathcafe.com

For information on supporting the dying in a holistic way
www.hospiceoftheheart.com

Grieving the loss of a loved one

When my mum died it felt as if the umbilical cord to all I was
had died with her. I wondered "who am I without her?" I felt
lost and abandoned. Even though I had been caring for her
for two years and had gone through a lot of anticipatory grief,
even though I was able to help her have a dignified death, I felt
like a six year old who has only just realised that their mum
is not coming back.

Sobonfu Somé, who died in January 2017, was an inspirational teacher from Burkina Faso in West Africa whose

mission for many years was to teach the wisdom of her country to Westerners. She shared the way that her culture dealt with loss and always stressed the importance of allowing the grieving process to unfold. There are a number of YouTube videos of her speaking and teaching to be accessed online. In an article in the magazine *Alternatives* she wrote about how grieving could be accepted as a normal part of life, how no one ever asked her whether she was finished grieving. Rather people would ask her whether she had grieved enough.

As a society there are things we can do to assist healing. Sobunfu suggested that we accept our own and each other's grief. There could be grief rooms and shrines in public spaces where people can go to grieve. Communal grieving, through witnessing and acknowledgement allows us to experience a level of healing that is profoundly freeing and validating.

One key component of dealing with grief in a healthy way is to simply let it happen. Allow yourself to feel each emotion as it arises. There is no clear duration that grieving is supposed to last; "stages" can come and go and everyone will experience them differently. It is not unusual, after someone has died, especially when you were present at the time, to feel disconnected from people, yourself, places or things; to feel cast adrift.

Grief is a continuous journey of letting go to understand how to move forward into the new phase of our life without that individual being physically present. Let go of the idea of normality for a while. When one is in the midst of grief normal time flies out the window. It can feel as if you are out of time and place when you feel so bereft. It can feel like you are looking at life behind glass, as if in a dream. You may feel that you don't know what to do with yourself, feeling lost, alone. You may find yourself deeply questioning everything about your life. There is no wrong or right way to grieve, but be as gentle as you can with yourself, have compassion for your feelings of shock, loss, sadness, and anger.

When we are bereaved, in addition to our own grief, we may also be left with a widowed parent or elderly relative who may not want to go on living without their partner. Their loneliness and despair can affect us greatly at the time when we are struggling with our own loss. Please take care of yourself during this grieving process.

- Sleep when you can or need to, you may feel totally exhausted at times.
- Ensure you allow time and space for your own feelings.
- Talk about the death, your loved one, perhaps writing a letter to them may be meaningful for you.
- Don't forget to eat, it is easily done but your body will benefit from good nourishment and it will help you to maintain stamina for all the things you have to do.
- Reach out to family and friends, talk to a therapist or grief counsellor.
- Honour your feelings, let tears flow.

"What soap is for the body, tears are for the soul."

Jewish proverb

"Give sorrow words; the grief that does not speak whispers the oe'r fraught heart and bids it break."

William Shakespeare

Creating an altar

I have worked with bereaved families and partners for the past ten years offering spiritual counselling, ways to process grief, and ceremonies that honour this. I recommend creating an altar for your loved one to help you with your grieving process. Create a special space in your home as an altar to honour your lost loved one in whatever way feels right for you. It helps bring a point of focus for grief, forgiveness and hope. Most bereaved families may instinctively gather up photos of the lost one, artwork they may have created, items they may have used in hobbies, favourite articles of clothing, letters, cards, jewelry, recipes, treasured poems, prayers. Place whatever you think is appropriate on a table, mantelpiece or shelf. Place fresh flowers there, have a candle lit or fairy lights.

Making an altar helps you reconnect to your loved one, bringing them closer to you, giving a sense of safety and accessibility in the midst of great sorrow. Visit your altar when you feel the need to reconnect with him or her.

Playing music they loved can also help keep them alive in your heart.

Creating an *Ofrenda* altar

Consider putting together your own *Ofrenda* to honour your loved one on the traditional All Saints Day celebration. The altar created in the Hispanic tradition honours the dead on *El Dia de los Muertes*, "The Day of the Dead" (November the first and second, All Saints and All Souls day). Latin Americans celebrate "The Day of the Dead" joyfully, with emphasis on celebrating and honouring the lives of their deceased loved ones. They feel they are celebrating the continuation of life; their belief is not that death is the end, but rather the beginning of a new stage in life.

The *Ofrenda* is a decorated area or table that displays offerings to deceased souls to show appreciation and love for them. The following items are usually displayed.

- *Photos and statues*
  A photo of the departed loved one. Statues of religious patron saints are also common in hispanic cultures.
- *Food and drink*
  The deceased's favourite food and drinks and bread are set out. Water is also placed there, signifying purity and renewal.
- *Flowers*
  Flowers symbolise the brevity of life, and are arranged on the Ofrenda. The traditional flower is the Mexican marigold. Their pungent aroma is said to help guide the dead home.
- *Candles*
  Many candles can be found on the Ofrenda. The many different shapes, sizes and designs signify those who remain alive, those the dead have left behind.
- *Incense*
  Copal incense is used to help spirits find their way to this world. Copal is the traditional incense used in Mexican churches and homes.
- *Favourite items*
  Favourite items of the deceased are placed on the Ofrenda.

You may find comfort in this tradition just as those from Hispanic cultures have for centuries.

Transforming grief

During my mother's final weeks, when I was giving her healing, she said, "I think I should like to come back as a butterfly". It was a beautiful sentiment that stayed with me, one I shared with the rest of the family. On the day of her cremation, I was struggling terribly with the thought of her body being burnt. It was her wish, but somehow I could not bear the thought of this desecration of her body, as I saw it through the eyes of my own grief. But as the curtains closed around the coffin, a red admiral butterfly flew down in a shaft of sunlight and landed on the curtains at the point of closure. All the congregation witnessed this but only my family and I knew the depth of its true significance and the solace that the butterfly's visit brought.

As you move through your cocoon of grief, in your own time you will start to feel more connected to the present as well as the past. You will emerge into the sunlight. You will be changed but you will do more than just survive, you will start to live. The words I spoke at my mother's memorial, eight months after her death were as a gentle reminder to stay in the moment and connect with life once more.

Helpful organisations

Cruse Bereavement Care
Helps people understand their grief and cope with loss. As well as counselling and support it offers information and advice.
www.cruse.org.uk

The Bereavement Register
A service designed to remove the names and addresses of people who have died from databases and mailing files. You can register at:
www.the-bereavement-register.com/uk
Tel 0870 600 7222

National Association of Widows
Information and support for those who have been widowed. Provides a supportive social life and friendship network via local branches.
www.nawidows.org.uk
Tel 0845 838 2261

Moving forward

"Losing my loved one left a huge gap in my life, I didn't know what to do after all that caring, but becoming a volunteer in a hospital filled that gap and it felt so good to feel needed. Volunteering helped me through my grief, I made new friends and felt a part of life once more."

Annie, carer

Use your loss

Create lasting tributes to your loved one. Consider memorial sites, scholarships, plaques, scrapbooks, or charitable contributions to honour their memory. Plant a tree, a wildflower meadow, have a dedicated bench in their favourite place which others can enjoy.

Write a story, create a poem, or make a film. Share your loved one's unique story with family members and other caregivers. Perhaps it is something that could be shared in schools or on the internet so more people can appreciate the qualities of your loved one and be touched by them.

Use your knowledge to help another. Contact your local Alzheimer's Association, Age UK or hospice provider and ask them to pair you with a brand new caregiver.

BE AWARE

Your acts of care and connection sustained your loved one through a difficult and perhaps long passage. Sharing what you have learned, cultivating happiness, and finding new meaning can create a fitting finale to your caregiving journey.

"Who then can so softly bind up the wound of another as he who has felt the same wound himself"

Thomas Jefferson

Reference Sources

Relative Matters
Chris Moon-Willems
www.relativematters.org

Caroline J Benham
www.brightcopperkettles.co.uk

Alzheimer's Association
Late stage caregiving
http://www.alz.org/care/alzheimers-late-end-stag
e-caregiving.asp

Alzheimer's Society Canada
Suggestions for the late stage for family members and caregivers
http://www.alzheimer.ca/en/Living-with-dementia/
Caring-for-someone/Late-stage-and-end-of-life/For-
family-members-and-caregivers

Felicity Warner, *Soul Midwife's Handbook*, Hay House 2012

Cathe Gaskell, www.theresultsco.co.uk

8

How to Give Compassionate
End of Life Care

"To care for the dying is sacred work. Death shouldn't
be something we have to shield each other from, rather
it is something we should guide each other through. At
the end of a person's life it will be the love that they have
received that they will remember. Love in care
is what sustains us."

Amanda Waring, Heart of Care

Until the mid-20th century, most people died at home, with
their family and friends surrounding them. Death was an
accepted part of everyday life but since that time the "western"
relationship with death has changed so much. We live much
longer and most elders die in a hospital, hospice, or residential
care, rather than at home with the family.

As carers supporting people near end of life we need to help an older person maintain the best quality of life possible. We need to minimise their suffering be it physical, emotional or spiritual. We need to support them to have a loving, digni- fied and peaceful death wherever possible. Let us recognise that those who are ending their lives in the frailty of old age deserve the same care and attention as those who are begin- ning their lives in the vulnerability of infancy. As a society we can see this as a burden or an opportunity to re-inspire our humanity by sharing one of our greatest attributes; being able to give and receive love.

Just as we value the birth companion, so we should recog- nise the importance of the death companion's role, and your kind and compassionate approach at this time will truly make a difference.

CONSIDER

During your interaction with an older person near end of life ask your- self how it would affect your actions to know that a part of the elder knows, sees, hears, and feels everything that you do, no matter how unresponsive they seem. How would you adjust your behaviour? Think about this often when caring for the dying to remind you to be present and respectful, sensitive and heartfelt.

Supporting dignity in dying

Many older people worry about a loss of control or a loss of dignity as their physical abilities decline. We should recognize, as carers, that there is no "right" or "correct" way to die. But it's everybody's right to die with dignity.

There are many ways in which you can help support the dignity of an elder at end of life.

- Ensure that pain management is effectively attended to. Pain can strip someone of their dignity very quickly.
- Ensure they have a voice regarding their own process of dying.
- Address emotional and spiritual suffering.
- Respect their privacy and address personal care issues sensitively.
- Value who they are.
- Help them feel emotionally connected with others.
- Assist them to resolve personal affairs.
- Have access to spiritual sources for support.
- Maintain independence, choice and control at end of life when so much feels out of control during their dying process.
- Consider the environment where sensitive issues are approached or bad news must be broken. These conversations need to be out of earshot of others, in a quiet room, a faith room or in the privacy of their own room without others being present unless they so wish.
- Remember that their death is an intensely personal experience, influenced by their belief system and personal history, which must be respected.
- Help them live and die well according to their wishes.

Talking about end of life wishes

Be prepared to initiate discussions about an elder's wishes for their future care. It's important to approach the conversation in a way that allows dignity and affords them respect. Ask for permission to have the discussion in the first place. It's not easy to talk about death, but it's important to clarify the older person's wishes while they are of sound mind and able to share their wishes. Memory loss or dementia can make the conversation very difficult, so advance planning is critical (see www. aplaceformom.com). Sometimes an elder may have resistance the first time you approach them, but don't be afraid to try again at another time or ensure that the relatives are having this discussion. Decisions about hydration, breathing support, and other interventions should be consistent with the elder's wishes and advance directives.

The National Hospice and Palliative Care Organization advises that it is important to be a good listener when having a sensitive discussion with an older person. They should be allowed to set the pace of the conversation. It is recommended that they should be asked important questions about what treatment they would prefer and what they would like to happen when they die. This should include their spiritual concerns and where they would prefer to die when the time comes. See www.caringinfo.org.

You could consider asking the following questions.

- Who would you like to be with you?
- Is there anyone you would not like to be present?
- What are you frightened of?
- How can we help those fears?
- In your last hours would you like some favourite music playing, what would that be?
- What are you spiritual needs?
- What rites or prayers would you like?
- Would you like a religious figure to be present?
- Are you comfortable with someone holding your hand?
- Would you like to be touched or massaged, are there areas of you body that you do not want to be touched?

- Do you like to have make up applied?
- What would you like to be dressed in?
- Do you want to be resuscitated or given antibiotics if you have to go into hospital?
- Where would be your ideal place to die?

Read How to Care for a Loved One section.

Compassion in action

Compassionate care encompasses kindness, patience, respect, generosity, unconditional love. The qualities of compassion and empathy can transform ourselves as well as others, providing us with a vocational aspect to caring as we become unafraid to connect with our heart. When we act from compassion and love our actions will be effective, we will not act inappropriately we will be benefiting others through promoting kindness and understanding.

Dr. Elizabeth Kübler-Ross was a pioneer in near-death studies and the author of several books on the subject of death and how to help the dying. She also developed an analysis of the process of grieving as a series of stages, which has been very influential. There are many videos of her on YouTube. She believed that if someone sends out love to others, the reflection of that love will come back to them. This would be like shining a light in the darkness of the time and place where you are "whether in the sickroom of a dying patient, on the corner of a ghetto in Harlem, or in your own home".

"Compassion in action restores pathways to the heart of those we care for, but also provides a pathway for the healing and understanding of ourselves."

Amanda Waring

Compassionate care tips

- Of course the dying need appropriate physical pain control but they also need to feel heard, cared-for, understood, accepted, connected and emotionally safe.
- Many old people may fear being a burden and yet at the same time fear being abandoned. Even when an elder cannot speak or smile their need for companionship remains. The older person may no longer recognise you, but may find comfort from your touch, the sound of your voice, and may understand what you are saying.
- Speak gently and kindly telling them who you are, what you are doing, or who is coming to visit them. Let them know when you are leaving and why, and when you will be back. Many elders may be less responsive but are still able to hear after they are no longer able to speak, so talk as if he or she can hear. The Buddha is said to have expressed this awareness: "Whatever words we utter should be chosen with care for people will hear them and be influenced by them for good or ill".
- When helping with night time care try and leave the older person with a good night blessing, or a wish for a peaceful night, your words might be the last words they hear, so make sure they are kind and positive.
- Staying calm and attentive will create a soothing atmosphere, and communicating through sensory experiences such as touch or singing can be reassuring to an elder.
- Contacts with pets or trained therapy animals can bring pleasure and ease transitions for even the most frail.
- Surrounding an elder with pictures and mementoes, reading aloud from treasured books, playing music, giving hand massages, reminiscing, and recalling life stories

promote dignity and comfort all the way through life's final moments.

- The older person will often be drowsy so plan visits and activities for times when they will be at their most alert.
- Allow those you care for to express their emotions, do not always jump in and however well-meaning tell them not to cry or be sad or don't be angry. Emotional and indeed physical healing can occur through the expressions of emotions, censoring or stopping that natural flow can cause more harm than good. It is preferable to acknowledge the emotion of that individual with compassion and empathy. Even if you can't provide a solution to the circumstances you can offer what you know provides solace to that individual be it music, a hug, or a cup of tea (or something stronger).
- There may be a decreased need for food and fluids but still ensure there is food for pleasure rather than just to survive! Let the elder choose if and when to eat or drink. Ice chips, water, or juice may be refreshing if they can swallow. Keep the older person's mouth and lips moist with products such as glycerin swabs and lip balm.
- Ensure that breakthrough pain is anticipated and attended to promptly and that you recognise the nuances of pain expressed by the elder.

Breath of life

If breathing is laboured what can help is if the elder's body is turned to the side and pillows are placed beneath the head and behind the back. A cool mist humidifier may also help. Assessing someone's breathing can give us clues as to how they may be feeling, even if they are unable to communicate verbally. Do not underestimate the power of breath to calm, heal and cleanse the body.

You may find you can connect with a distressed elder by first copying their breathing patterns audibly yourself. Maintain eye contact and once you have made that connection and are breathing with their rhythm and volume gently slow your breath down to a more peaceful pace. Often this connecting and then slowing enables an elder to match their breathing to your calmer pace, almost by osmosis. Breathe together in this calmer place. Try and experiment with this as part of your communication skills with those near end of life or in pain at any stage. For more breathing techniques go to www.holotropic.com.

"I would like to learn some breathing techniques, because I am really anxious and fearful about not being able to catch my breath at the end. I saw my mum struggle terribly and I can't get that out of my mind at times."

Theresa, carer

Physical care tips at end of life

There may be a loss of bladder or bowel control so keep the older person as clean, dry, and comfortable as possible. Discreetly place disposable pads on the bed beneath the elder and remove them regularly when they become soiled. It is important to have an elder maintain personal hygiene for comfort levels and the prevention of infection.

Washing

Do

- be gentle with the presence of sores;
- rinse soap off completely and dry skin gently;

- ensure the water is changed several times during the wash;
- add moisturising creams gently and to the soles of the feet;
- use wet wipes if the older person prefers this.

Mouth care

Most people who are dying have mouth problems, ulcers, bleeding gums, excess saliva, altered taste. Relieve a dry mouth with ice cubes, frozen fruit, lemonade or tonic water. Tinned unsweetened pineapple can help. A soft baby toothbrush is best if the older person's mouth is sore. Only use a small amount of toothpaste, peppermint and fluoride may be too strong, try fennel or calendula.

Emotional care tips at end of life

As a carer you can offer emotional comfort in many ways, but the most important gift you can give to a dying person is to listen. You may find this kind of emotional intimacy daunting at times, but just breathe slowly, calm yourself and listen from your heart.

Do

- Recognise that anger at end of life is a common reaction, be aware that there may be yelling, agression or hostility but allow the older person to express their fears around their death. This may come in waves of guilt, sadness, recrimination, bitterness, despair, helplessness. Listen actively and with an open heart, ensure you have details of professionals, counsellors, pastoral care that may help. Consider asking them if they would like to speak with a specific person about these fears.

- Recognise that as palliative care increases and a feeling of dependency increases too, that an elder may feel overwhelmed with inadequacy or embarrassment at the intimate changes that may be happening for them. Reassure them that you are with them, not judging them in any way. Be extra sensitive around intimate discussions regarding loss of bodily functions and the consequences.

- Recognise the fears that come up around being in pain and discomfort. Reassure them that pain will be contained and that you will not let it become out of control. Ensure you have the right medications for this and anticipate breakthrough pain in advance.

- Recognise that talking about their own past is another way some elders gain perspective on their life and the process of dying.

- Recognise that many older people prefer to be included in discussions about issues that concern them. Do not withhold information unless specifically directed to by them.

- Recognise that elders need reassurance that you will honour their wishes and ensure that wills and advance directives are followed through according to their requests. Reassure them that they can trust you to follow through.

- Recognise that any outstanding issues, emotional or financial, can cause stress to the elder and find ways to resolve issues with them as much as possible.

- Recognise that dying can feel very lonely and frightening for some, so take time to watch movies together, read, talk, sing to them or simply sit and hold their hand.

- Recognise that even at end of life new precious memories can be made, and your love and care may be part of them.

Spiritual care tips

- Never force your own faith and beliefs onto another.
- Always respect the spiritual/religious creeds of another.
- You might like to find some prayers in keeping with the dying person's tradition. These could also include psalms, poems and extracts from spiritual books.
- Ask the elder if there are any religious ceremonies or rituals that they would like prior to death.
- Would they like singing, chanting, poems or prayers spoken out loud? Instruments such as drums and bells are used in many traditions at this time. The sounds of nature can be very healing.
- Would they like to be anointed or to receive healing or any other therapies close to death?
- Who would they like to have with them or not to have with them?

BE AWARE

Remember to provide plenty of opportunities for people to continue to grow emotionally and spiritually. Whilst someone is still breathing they are still feeling, growing, loving. Do not focus so much on their dying that you forget their living. Pleasure, love, surprise, delight are gifts to share and inspire.

"I want something to look forward to
I want a carer to support my faith needs
I want to laugh and be surprised
I never want a carer to destroy my sense of hope
I may be dying but I can still enjoy ice cream"

Hazel, eighty-eight

"I was visiting a Hospice, in the company of a colleague who acted as consultant to them, and the staff were upset about a dying train driver, a life-long trade unionist, who was effing and blinding his way to death. The staff were feeling they had failed in not getting a quiet acceptance; I suggested that he was dying as he had lived – fighting his corner to the end and that was true to him, and not their failure."

Barbara Dearnley, retired nurse

Connecting

We need to understand the importance of maintaining relationships and developing connections. Encourage friends and families to make an informal picture book with old and new memories interspersed with written memories and experiences and how that dying person has shaped and inspired their lives. It then becomes something you can share over again with the elder when they are lonely or feeling that their life had little impact.

You can use storylane.com or storycorps.org onto which relatives record memories and family stories. You can try thinkingofyou.com to post a story of gratitude in written or videotaped form. You can use voicequilt.com to invite family and friends to record messages on a free voice message system where elders can then listen to the messages on line.

Use music as medicine

Our human bodies are like musical instruments, our heart beating within provides our sacred rhythm. The power of sound to heal and harmonise is well documented and prescriptive live music played to the dying, known as music-thanatology can inspire, motivate, soothe, and ease pain symptoms. Elders respond more directly and deeply (even when unconscious) to the sounds of the harp when played live at the bedside as they do to the voice and this is a wonderful gift to provide for the elders in your care. For more info go to www.apmt.org or www.bsmt.org

Singing together produces a wonderful feeling of cama-raderie whether the songs are carols, lullabies, hymns or any other kind of song that may inspire or bring comfort. Listen to different types of music that can create an atmosphere of peace or joy or whatever is appropriate to support the emotional needs of those in your care. You can be their spiritual DJ and compile the music on an iPad or something similar.

Leaving a legacy

At the end of life many older people may want to reflect on the story of their life, and how they lived it, needing to feel that their life has had meaning. It's important that you listen sensitively and with empathy. During these conversations you could ask them what they feel most proud of, their most important accomplishments. You could ask them what lessons they have learned from life that they might like to pass on to you or others. They may wish to leave something behind for their loved ones: guidance; advice; or even instructions for their family; to help them prepare for the future. They may want to leave a creative reminder for loved ones. You can help them with this by offering assistance with creating their legacy. Some ideas include:

- lockets with pictures;
- leaving a diary;
- making memory boxes;
- devising recipe books;

- making recordings such as reading nursery rhymes for grandchildren;
- creating a book of their wisdom, favourite jokes, happiest memories;
- putting pictures and keepsakes from favourite holidays into a scrap book;
- creating digital slideshows, photo, or other albums;
- recording and writing songs;
- poems and recordings of them speaking their favourite poems;
- paintings, drawings, sketches, illustrations;
- making embroidered cushions, or book marks;
- creating plaster casts of their hands;
- making rings with their thumb print on them;
- fabric painting t-shirts and scarves.

You can use storylane.com or storycorps.org to create digital legacies.

Forgiveness and building bridges

When people are nearing death, there is often a deep need to confront and resolve unfinished issues from their past, particularly with family members. One of the most important things you can do as a carer for those near end of life is to provide opportunities for the mending of broken or troubled relationships. Regrets about what one might have done, could have done, should have done may surface quite dramatically for older people when they are faced with life threatening illness. Gentle empathetic and emotional skills are needed to guide them through the mire of self- recrimination, guilt and loss.

As death approaches, an older person may confide about their past and ask for forgiveness. They may wish to see someone to make amends while they still can. If it is not possible to get the person to the bedside you could help the older person make a recorded message and get it sent on for them. One of the most common causes of grief is not having the opportunity to tell someone that you love them before they die, or not hearing from them that they love you. Provide opportunities for this to happen, through Skype, video, letters, email. Help the older person have a more peaceful death, and keep them connected to loved ones where possible.

End of life care for elders with dementia

At this stage an elder will be confined to bed and dependent on you for all personal care. They will need you to advocate, connect, and attend to their physical and emotional needs. Even when those with dementia have progressed to the end of life stage, meaningful engagement remains possible through sensory based activity and interaction, although the person may no longer be able to verbalise their appreciation of the benefit.

- Try giving a hand and foot massage using a loving touch to aid relaxation.
- Carefully brush or comb the person's hair with slow movements to help them feel soothed and cared for.
- Gently move their arms and legs to music to help keep their limbs flexible.
- Spray their pillow with a favourite scent to lift the atmosphere or bring fresh scented flowers in bloom into their room or warming winter scents of cinnamon and pine.
- Bring the unexpected into their space, blow some bubbles, wear an extraordinary hat connecting with them through gentle humour.

- Read a favourite story to them or loved poems or letters or emails from loved ones. Sing lullabies.
- Play a recording of birdsong or their favourite music.
- Ensure you keep bright sun off their face.
- Dim the lights and consider bringing in battery operated colour changing candles.
- Offer nourishment and beverages throughout the day. This continuous hydration approach has decreased, and in some cases eliminated, urinary tract infections.
- You may find it difficult to understand what they are saying or what they may want but research has highlighted many instances of those with severe dementia suddenly becoming lucid enough to say farewell to those around them, or talk coherently about seeing dead relatives. So do not dismiss what they say as disjointed ramblings.

"When my dad who had Alzheimer's was dying he recovered sufficiently to have a day of complete clarity when we were able to say all we needed to say. It was wonderful, so unexpected, a miracle and I feel ready to move forward now"

Abigail, carer

Pain management

Managing pain and discomfort requires frequent monitoring and reassessment of subtle nonverbal signals. Slight behavioural changes can signal unmet needs. Communicating written observations, times, and events will provide valuable clues about the elder's pain status. Ensure pain assessment charts are up to date and if the patient's pain is worsening considerably don't delay, report it to the relevant person immediately and record it on the chart later.

Keep your connection to that elder, do not leave them on their own because they now seem "no bother". They still need your attentive care, more than ever perhaps. The soothing properties of touch, massage, music, fragrance, and a loving voice can also reduce pain. Be open to trying different approaches and observe the elder's reactions.

"I stood outside his room and heard him scream in pain when they changed him. I asked for the morphine to be increased and was told that this would result in him being semi-conscious. I couldn't see why this was a problem. There seemed to be difficulty in understanding that my father should be nursed appropriately for a dying person rather than someone who would recover. You wouldn't treat animals like this leaving them in pain, it broke my heart."

David, carer

BE PREPARED

Ensure that the relatives understand that with certain strong pain relief at end of life, their loved one may slip into a coma. Therefore any important conversations need to be had before this happens. Poor communication around this has left many relatives in deep grief, denied the opportunity to say their final goodbyes.

Supporting the relatives

Provide sensitive support for family members and loved ones. Those with relatives with dementia have witnessed their loved one go to the brink of death and back again often many times, they may be exhausted from this constant preparation to let

go. Many relatives may have battled to make difficult treatment, placement, and intervention choices for their loved ones
whilst struggling with the pain of loss and guilt. Be gentle and
respectful to relatives, recognise their pain and ask how you
may help them. Respect the rights of families and elders who
refuse treatments.

End of life experiences

We should allow the space for those we care for to share their
experiences of the "unexplainable". These could be seeing
angels, coloured orbs, deceased loved ones or pets. They may
say these apparitions have come to collect them or help them
let go. If it is something that brings them comfort and strength
then just acknowledge how lovely this is for them. Tell them
how much it means to you to know that they are receiving
reassurance even if you are unable to share their visions. Put
any prejudice or disbelief to one side and truly listen. Help
them by asking questions such as: "What does he/she look
like?; How many have come to visit you?; What are they
saying?; What does it look like, or feel like?". Do not dismiss
these other worldly spiritual experiences for they will be very
real for that individual.

When my granny was dying she kept seeing coloured lights
everywhere, but unthinking staff kept telling her that there
was nothing there, she was just seeing things. This made my
granny fearful and she worried for her sanity at end of life
rather than feeling comforted. There is a clear difference
between such visions and drug induced hallucinations, which
can include seeing the wall paper moving, insects crawling
up the walls, floors moving and weird creatures walking. If
the elder is experiencing the latter they may shiver or pluck at
their sheets. Evidence that these disconcerting hallucinations

are happening should be reported so that medication can be given to help control them and relax and soothe the person.

In contrast, those who have spiritual end of life experiences mainly seem to be calmed and soothed by them. Research has shown that end of life visions and dreams hold profound meaning for the dying and actually help them to come to terms with the dying process. They may talk about other worldly realms or embarking on a journey, or turn towards the window and experience a sudden sense of wonder and joy.

"Oh wow, oh wow, oh wow"
                                   Last words, Steve Jobs, CEO Apple

Those who witness end of life experiences often describe them as beautiful, comforting and readying. So allow room for the mystery of life and death without judging or correcting the experiences of others. It is not for us to say whether it is authentic or imagined, who knows what we may see or feel when our time comes.

Being with the dying

I have sat with the dying since I was eight years old, when I used to be taken by my granny to sing at the bedside of those who were terminally ill in the hospitals where she volunteered. Even at such a young age I seemed to have an understanding of what was needed through sound and songs, or holding that person's hand. It was as if I had done it before. I was not frightened. As a teenager I continued to sing regularly to those in the Royal Hospital and Home for Incurables, as it was then called, and in other care homes, to help bring comfort and ease to elders in their final days. From my twenties onwards

I have undertaken many trainings and initiations in shamanism, Celtic ways, Hawaiian healing, Buddhist meditation and Native American rites of passage, to assist the transition of those who are dying. I instinctively use this knowledge when working in my role as death doula, or soul midwife, and it is an absolute privilege to do this work. In this section I will be sharing some of the ways I use to help support a person as they leave this world behind.

All around the world communities have their own specific traditions for sitting with, and keeping watch over, those who are dying. This is often known as a Vigil. Everyone's death is unique and the purpose of sitting with the dying is to honour their experience and nurture it by giving them all our attention, kindness and care. So if possible be open to being with the dying, as sharing part of their journey with them can actually be one of life's most enriching experiences.

"I think the hardest thing for a caregiver is just to Be, without having to fix anything, or change anything or move someone along through the stages so that they feel more comfortable."

Sally

When you as a carer have the opportunity to sit with the dying you can bring in peace and compassion, just allow yourself to be. You may find this to be an extremely sacred time, even if you only have ten minutes to spare. Always introduce yourself and say when you are leaving. Remember that hearing will be present until the end, so never assume the person will be unable to hear you. Talk as if they can hear you. Strong physical contact can be painful or too invasive, so it is best to sit beside the bed and gently hold their hand or stroke them with a gentle touch. Even when a person is unconscious or semi-conscious they might be able to respond with faint pressure from their thumb.

You can help to create a safe, protected and beautiful space for them during this time. If you feel inclined to you can bless this space each time you enter or leave. I say or sing the words that I wrote for the very purpose of creating a sacred space around a dying person. I create a dedicated peaceful space for that person's passing, which can often feel anything but, as there may be call bells going off, staff talking noisily, cries from other older residents or patients and noisy machines. The effect of the words spoken or sung can make the room feel calm, protected and the elder more peaceful.

> *By the grace of your grace*
> *you have made this a sacred space*
> *by the grace of your grace you have.*
> *By the grace of your grace*
> *you have made this a sacred place*
> *by the grace of your grace you have.*
> *Oh thank you, oh thank you*
> *Oh thank you, oh thank you*
> *By the grace of your grace we are ONE*
> *or*
> *By the grace of your grace it is done.*
> **Amanda Waring**

The recording of my singing this and other of my songs and meditations are available for you to use. My CD *I Am Near You* has soothing melodies and words to help calm and uplift and bless those who are dying.

See amandawaring.com and amandawaringevents.com

Creating a peaceful environment

Lower the lighting until it is soft or bring in battery operated candles, or fairy lights. Try to keep bright sunlight away from their face and eyes. Create a peaceful, soothing atmosphere by playing a favourite piece of music or inviting a music thanatologist in to play live at the bedside. Consider reading a spiritual passage or religious text that means something to that older person. If appropriate arrange for end of life prayers to be said by a chaplain, vicar, priest or other faith ministers.

Perhaps the bed could be moved so that they can see the sky or nature. You might consider hanging wind chimes or rainbow catchers in the window. A bird feeder near the window could also provide an interest and a sense of connection with nature.

Make the room smell as lovely as possible by using an incense diffuser, aromatherapy oils, or bringing in flowers. You might like to spritz their pillow with their favourite scent or the room with an aromatherapy spray. As much as seventy-five per cent of our emotions are thought to be generated by what we smell, so use aromas sensitively to bring an atmosphere of peace, freshness and tranquility. However be aware that when people are dying their sensitivity to odours can be acute so if there is any negative reaction remove fragrances immediately.

Try and counter the sterility of, or medical aspect to, their environment. Place a beautiful throw on their bed for colour, style and comfort. Place photos of loved ones or religious figures appropriate to their faith near them, or you may consider setting up an altar for them.

Do ensure there are extra tissues and water glasses for relatives who may be visiting.

When someone is in the dying process

"This can often be a slow and gentle unravelling almost like the labour before the birth."

**Felicity Warner, author and founder
of the Soul Midwives movement**

Emotionally there are three phases that may occur in the dying process. The first is a feeling of emotional chaos once there is an acknowledgement that death is happening. After this time of fighting and resisting comes a point of surrender, and accepting the flow of the inevitable process. Finally, a feeling of bliss or even joy occurs very briefly as the last transition takes place. There are certain indicators that let us know when someone has tipped into the dying process.

- There can be physical changes, teeth can discolour or develop dark stains. The body of the person may shrink in stature and skin can become paper thin.
- There can be a slow withdrawal from wanting to take part in conversations, interactions and an unwillingness to get out of bed.
- They may yawn more, even when unconscious, as this is a natural response allowing more oxygen to be drawn into the body.
- They may express gratitude to carers and relatives in preparation for final goodbyes.
- They may begin to refuse visits from friends and relatives and seek the company of just one or two people.
- They may feel uncomfortable, asking to be repositioned more often, or complaining that the pillows are not comfy. The room temperature may feel too hot or too cold. They will feel more sensitive to noise.

- They may often mumble, reach out for invisible objects, laugh, twitch, make jerking movements or cry out.
- They will sleep more for long periods and drift in and out of consciousness.
- They may have liquid that gathers in the throat and chest resulting in an unpleasant sound called a death rattle. This is normally not distressing to the dying person.
- They may talk about "leaving" or making some kind of journey.
- They may be fearful, or confide in you about their past and ask for forgiveness.

Pacifying fears

Often I have heard relatives say to me "I've told Mum she is not to talk to me about her death, I can't bear it, it will just make it happen quicker". Who then does that elder have to turn to with their concerns and fears? It could be you. Allow yourself to be open to supporting in this way and to indeed find ways of pacifying your own fears around death. You can use a soft approach in an indirect way to the older person by asking, "I wonder if there's anything you want to talk to me about?" You could also ask, "What can I do to help you at the moment?" Or perhaps you could say, "If there ever comes a time when you want to talk about something or you feel frightened, please do tell me or let me find someone for you". This gives the elder permission to talk in his, or her, own time, without expectations being placed on them.

If the elder has fears, encourage them to share them, you might not be able to resolve them but at least they can be heard and witnessed by you. This will help to lay them to rest and bring some peace to that elder.

*

"We work not to provide answers but friendship, to share not to solve. We bring no one but ourselves and that is our greatest gift."

Richard Allen, author and educator

Night presents the greatest challenges; anxiety is always highest in the small hours. So make sure to find out from the elder or relatives what gives them strength when they are in the depths of despair, and how they call on it. Armed with this knowledge when anxious or challenging times arise you can help them reconnect to their sources of courage. Ensure this is in the care plan.

Ask the elder if they would like a picture of a spiritual figure or guide near them by their bed if they have indicated this is in keeping with their faith and hope needs. They may like a picture of Jesus, Buddha, Krishna, Mother Mary. If they do not have one you could perhaps organise that one be printed from the internet. Repeating or chanting the name of an individual's God, angel or ally has been found to bring strength and comfort.

A common fear for someone who is dying is the fear of the unknown. "Where do I go when I die?", they may wonder, especially if they are a person who does not have a strong faith or belief system. They can be worrying that they may just be going into never ending darkness, a dark black hole.

Guided imagery to help anxiety

One way you can help the person close to death relieve this anxiety is to use the power of imagery to help them create a peaceful journey to a place where they can imagine resting after death. Imagination is one of our most powerful inner resources and using this power we can move away from fearful images, replacing them with loving and calming images. Guided imagery can be an effective and comforting tool for decreasing fear, anxiety and pain. It is something I use often with the dying; as I take them on the mental journey I can see elders following their imagination and pacifying their fears. Below is an example of how I lead someone through this form of visualisation and I hope you might consider sharing something similar.

Recognise that in our lives we go through many transitions, from leaving our mother's womb, through to saying goodbye to childhood as we become an adult. Throughout our lives we are continually moving through life events, embracing changes, releasing, growing, learning, shedding old patterns, the past, re-adjusting, moving through, loving, leaving, loving, feeling, breathing, letting go. A life of change and death, birth and growth, grief and wonder, trust and love ... and now there is another transition, a letting go to a place where you can feel held, protected, peaceful and loved ... a place that is yours, a place that we can visit now and return to again and again.

So imagine you are standing at a beautiful wrought iron gate that you can push gently open to reveal an enticing woodland grove, your woodland grove. The sun is shining through the leaves, dappling dancing light shines upon an inviting pathway lined with bluebells. The smell is delicious as you walk amongst the swathes of gorgeous nodding bluebells, they seem to be almost welcoming you.

You follow the gentle meandering path, delightful birdsong serenading you as you walk beneath the trees, feeling the loving warmth of the sun and delighting in the sights and smells around you. The path opens up to a wild flower meadow filled with flowers of every colour, quite breath taking, you walk through this sea of colour to the centre of the meadow where on a raised grassy mound you come upon a most inviting seat. You take off your shoes, feeling the soft cooling grass ▶

beneath your feet, and you walk over to this extremely comfortable seat, so relaxed, so at peace, all is well, all is well, all is well. You can stay here as long as you wish, listening to the bird song, resting, feeling peaceful.

The seat is long enough for you to lie down if you like, and you gaze upwards to the blue sky above as the golden rays of the sun gently warm your skin. All is well, and all is well, and all is well as you are bathed in sunlight and listen to the sounds of nature around you. You find yourself speaking words softly to yourself. I am unfurling, uncurling, basking in the sun, my shadow is no more, my soul is at one with the love and the peace that this blessed light brings and my joyous heart remembers, remembers and sings . . . I am home, I am home, I am home. Almost as an echo to your words you feel a presence of a Being, a loved one, a guide perhaps. You feel the benediction from their presence, their healing, compassion and grace. They take your hands in theirs and with infinite tenderness offer you this blessing.

Infinite grace and gentleness, be upon you.
infinite purity and peace be within you.
infinite wisdom and wellness guide you.
Infinite harmony and happiness delight you.
Infinite goodness and gratitude be with you.
infinite light and love surround you.
infinite life of love bless you.

Feeling full of light and love you express your heartfelt thanks, say your goodbyes and gently and peacefully walk back upon the inviting path that leads you through the meadow and the bluebells beneath the trees to the intricate wrought iron gate. You take one last look at your special place, knowing you will return again whenever you need to. Now gently push through the gate and return slowly in your own time to the here and now.

Sometimes people fall asleep during this, becalmed and peaceful, which is so lovely to see.

Dark night of the soul

For most people during the final dying stages there can be a passage of time which is commonly known as "the dark night of the soul". It can be the lowest point for the person in the pre-death stage and it can sometimes last for days. This time can seem to echo the feelings of rejection and heartbreaking vulnerability that Jesus expressed when he was dying on the cross. This can be the stage when even the most spiritual or religious people temporarily lose their faith and feel utterly abandoned and often very fearful.

As a carer recognise that this stage is common near end of life and reassure the elder that they will move through this. For indeed they do. You can use something similar to my guided imagery or write your own to help them. Stay with them where you can so that they can feel the comfort of your presence.

Felicity Warner, author of *Gentle Dying* and *The Soul Midwives' Handbook*, is the founder of the Soul Midwives movement. For her there is a link between this time and the final act of surrender. The decision must be made to let go and trust and to allow the ego to dissolve. There seems to be a specific period close to the point of death when the person who is dying "must detach from all comforting belief systems". This for them is "an utterly desolate experience" but when they come out of it they have no more fear and it is "as if they are standing in the sun".

Whilst some elders may question their spiritual or religious beliefs at this time, others may find solace in an old or new faith. During this phase I will often say either out loud or silently, "Peace be with you, upon you and around you". I imagine them held in a circle of golden light, or envisage loving arms around them, or angels' wings. I may play music or sing to them. I may anoint their feet, and hands and fore-head with some beautiful frankincense oil.

I may read prayers from their faith or others in hope of bringing them comfort. Please search for ones that will be right for that individual based on your knowledge of them, their religion and their responses. I have used Vedic hymns, ancient Indian proverbs and Tibetan meditations when they seemed appropriate, there are many other sources to draw on.

The prayer called the Saint Francis prayer is very popular and is one I like to use to give hope. Although it is often assumed that Saint Francis wrote it and it is the kind of thing he might have written, he was not the author. Nobody actu-ally knows who did write it, the text was first published in France in 1912.

Saint Francis Prayer

> *Lord, make me an instrument of Your peace.*
> *Where there is hatred, let me sow love;*
> *where there is injury, pardon;*
> *where there is doubt, faith;*
> *where there is despair, hope;*
> *where there is darkness, light;*
> *where there is sadness, joy.*
>
> *O, Divine Master, grant that I may not so much seek to be*
> *   consoled as to console;*
> *to be understood as to understand;*

to be loved as to love;
For it is in giving that we receive;
it is in pardoning that we are pardoned;
it is in dying that we are born again to eternal life.

I find that the words of Psalm 23 'The Lord is my shepherd' can give comfort. I also draw inspiration from Father Damien, who worked for many years with lepers in Molokai in Hawaii, eventually contracting the disease himself. He has been recognised by a saint by the Catholic church. He did not see death as something to be feared but to be welcomed because it is the messenger of God. "It is the last and the greatest of God's gifts."

I have written my own poem to bring peace to the heart of the one who is leaving.

May there be peace in the east
and peace in the west
may there be peace in the north
and peace in the south
may there be peace within
and peace without
and may your journey of peace begin.
Amanda Waring, 2016

Letting go

When I work with the dying near the very last stages it feels appropriate, indeed there is almost an instinctive urge, to give permission for that individual to go. At this time soul midwives will perhaps whisper in that person's ear, saying they can follow the light and be greeted by someone who has come to help them and who loves them. I may soothe and calm them by repeating their name softly and saying all is well, they are doing so well, they can gently let go. Then at this time I might say the following words.

Wings of love surround you, you are held tenderly, loved so, blessed so, knowing all this, you can let go. Held in love and blessed be, you are held in the unity of all that it is and all that was and all that is to be. The breath of peace reminds you to softly leave this place, to move freely into your space of divine grace, loved for evermore on the other shore.

Amanda Waring, *I am Near You* **CD**

I might use another poem that I have written to encourage the soul to fly free.

> *You are a fledgling leaving a nest*
> *a nest you have outgrown*
> *it seems like all you have known,*
> *but there is another world for you to explore*
> *a world where you will find*
> *you are adored*
> *open your wings and let*
> *your spirit soar*
> *you can fly across your soul's sky*
> *loved and free.*
> *take that leap and you'll see*
> *you will find your way home to me.*

Amanda Waring, 2017

Tip – I use beautiful music to ease letting go. I recommend One Hundred Thousand Angels, Bliss records, Lynne Morrison, Cave of Gold, Greentrax recording, the chants of the Ceile De www.ceilede.co.uk.

Helping an elder let go of the physical body

I help the elder let go of the physical body with honour, gratitude and understanding for all that this body has allowed them to do. Some elders may have a sense of disgust for, or disappointment in, their body, feeling that it is letting them down. They may not like the way it looks, feels or smells. You can help them address this by acknowledging the gift that body has been in their lifetime. I do this by taking them through a body blessing ceremony.

I take their hands in mine and say . . .

Bless these wonderful hands, these hands that have given so much, shared so much, held and stroked your loved ones, and pets. Hands that have tended to your garden, cooked delicious meals, allowed you to paint, write, draw, connect. Bless these hands that have given you the gift of being able to make, create, feel, cherish and love. Bless these incredible beautiful hands.

Next I would go down to gently touch their feet and say . . .

Bless these amazing feet, these feet that have given you the ability to dance and run and jump. These feet that have carried you to loved ones, allowed you to explore this earth, feel the cool grass beneath them, the warm sand, and paddle in refreshing water. These feet that have given you the gift of travel, connection and freedom. Bless these beautiful feet.

Then I would go to gently touch their forehead and say . . .

Bless this extraordinary mind, this mind that has let you learn, absorb, read, teach and share so much knowledge. This mind that has helped and influenced the minds of others and problem solved and found solutions. Bless the gift of your mind that has passed on so much understanding to others.

Next I would lightly let my hand hover over their heart, not touching this time and say . . .

Bless this amazing heart, this heart that has felt so much, loved so much, shared so much, healed so much, held so much, bless this incredible beautiful heart.

Finally I would go back to holding their hands and saying . . .

Bless your whole physical being for the journey you have taken together and with gratitude to your physical form we can gently say let go, let go, let go.

You may be more comfortable with just holding that elder's hands and saying simply, "What a gift these hands have been to others, how much love they have given, isn't that wonderful".

A simple recognition can suffice and ease the transition.

"I felt my mum was hanging on so I said to her that we would miss her so, but she had given us so much that we would manage, she was not to worry. We all love you, you will never be forgotten but if it's time for you to go, our love travels with you."

Tara, carer

"When God calls you no matter where you are, Timbuktu, Africa, another country, you just have to go. I have no fear of death whatsoever."

Robert, carer

What happens physically when a person dies

The breath is very important as many cultures have recognised. All our lives we breathe in and out and then in death we breathe no more.

your breath moves in and out
we have a rhythm and a way
inherent in our lives every day

but in the stilling and the quiet
a new way of being emerges,
it urges one to move and flow
out of what was, into the eternal now,
feel that rhythm, that call, as soft and as precious
as anything you have known
and let go . . . .

Amanda Waring, 2017

Always make a note of the time of death. In the UK the death must be certified and registered and the body must be disposed of in accordance with the births and deaths registration act 1926.

When a person dies:

- the heart stops beating, breathing stops, the body colour becomes pale;
- the body cools, muscles relax, urine and stools may release;
- the eyes may remain open;
- the jaw can fall open but cloths wrapped around their head and jaw can ensure their jaw stays closed before rigormortis sets in;
- the trickling of internal fluids may be heard;
- there can be a sense that they are just "not home" anymore;
- they may look very peaceful.

Speak quietly and behave respectfully around the person who has died. Silence noisy machines, dim the lights, reduce all controllable noises, put pagers and phones on vibrate.

Maria Dancing Heart is a hospice counsellor. In her book

Last Adventure of Life, published by Findhorn Press, she
explains the policy at the hospice where she works. There,
the staff encourage families to remain with the body of
their loved one as long as they need to. She describes one
situation where, while the family was gathering, a son went
on reading to his mother. He was reading from a book she
had asked him to read to her at the end of her life, a book
incidentally that she thought it would benefit her son to
read. This ritual, comments Maria, "reminded me of the
Tibetan Buddhist ritual, in which a person from the temple
comes to read to the deceased soul from the *Tibetan Book of
the Dead* for as many as forty-nine days". Tibetan Buddhists
believe that even after death the soul is able to hear for this
period.

Post mortem care

This needs to be done promptly, quietly, efficiently, with
dignity and compassion. If you have been very close to that
elder this part of the care may seem like an honour or it may
be very emotional for you. You may never have seen a dead
body and some people can feel shocked or frightened so please
seek support and assistance, be gentle with yourself and the
elder that has passed. Do what you can do and for what you
can't, get the help you need.

After the pronouncement of death
Respect the body. I believe the dead have the right to gentle,
careful treatment. It is important to care for the person who
has died as if their family or friends were standing beside us.
Remember the deceased had a name in life, and they have a
name in death, and this is how you should refer to them.

CONSIDER having that person's favourite piece of music playing in the background as you work on the body.

Below is a list of procedures that will need to be carried out and some suggestions as to how to go about them.

- Remove tubes.
- Replace soiled dressings.
- Pad anal area.
- Gently wash the body to remove discharge if appropriate.
- Place the elder on their back with head and shoulders elevated.
- Grasp the eyelashes and gently pull the lids down.
- Insert dentures as soon as possible before *rigor mortis* sets in.
- Place a clean gown, or whatever clothing was requested by the individual, on the body. Cover with a sheet unless requested not to.
- Place flowers or an object of personal significance for that individual, perhaps a photo or a locket, in the hands. Flowers can be placed on the eyelids too and petals around and on the body.
- Follow any specific requests about this moment.
- You may feel you wish to open the window, a tradition in some cultures.
- You may want to say your own words and blessings for the departed.
- Keep the place where the elder's body is as peaceful and restful as possible.
- Tend to your own grief.
- Gently notify family members. You need to have found

out who wants to be called about the death. Do they want to be woken up, do they want someone with them, who do they want to tell them?

- Prepare the paperwork for the removal of the body.
- Respectfully gather eyeglasses and belongings. Ensure there are lovely carriers, bags, suitcases, decorated boxes for you to put the elder's things into, as it is awful for a relative to find their loved ones belongings in black bin bags, as if the person that had died was now just being thrown out with the rubbish. Fold clothes neatly and with care. You may wish to write or leave a personal message with them.

"I had not seen a dead body before. I was anxious and nervous but found my courage and approached my father's body. As I came close I felt a voice, not heard it exactly but felt it whispered within me. It was my father's voice saying, 'I am alright, I am OK, I love you'. I just knew it was dad and this has given me strength and comfort and completely removed my fear of dying."

Lou, carer

Salvatore Gencerelle, author of *Man Among the Helpers*, spent seventeen years under the supervision of a Native American healer. He has written that the modern world has "become unable to accept the gift that death provides". We no longer remember that death is the final rite of passage and the "return to the great mystery".

Requirements and beliefs of different faiths and cultures

All religious traditions offer various rituals to help us cope with end of life transitions. Whatever your tradition may be, or indeed whichever tradition you most relate to, tailor those rituals to your need, and find comfort and solace in them. There is much healing to be found in the practice of rituals when dealing with death and grief. Here is a short summary of the beliefs, rituals and requirements of different faiths.

BUDDHISM

Buddhists believe that when they die they will be born again. They seek to escape the cycle of birth and death and rebirth to attain *Nirvana*, the state of total peace. At the time of death specific chants and prayers may be recited. The body should be left for three days following a death and the *Bardo* practice may be offered for forty-nine days after death.

HINDUISM

Hindus believe in reincarnation. Death to them is the process of the soul moving closer to heaven (*Nirvana*). If possible, at the time of death a Hindu should be lying on the floor in order to have contact with the earth. Any physical touching of the body is frowned upon other than by certain relatives who will pray around the body soon after death has occurred.

ISLAM

Shi'ite and Sunni Muslims accept death as the will of Allah and acknowledge and prepare for their death with daily prayers. Many Muslims believe that by accepting Islam and saying the *Shahadah*, their declaration of faith, they will reach *Jannah*, (heaven) after death. Often a dying person from this faith may wish to face Mecca. The body should be buried within twenty-four hours of death and turned to face Mecca. Family members or friends will perform the ritual washing and wrap the body in a shroud. Females wash females and males wash males.

JUDAISM

Jews believe that when they die they join God in heaven, which is called *Olam HaEmet*, the World of Truth. They acknowledge death as part of God's plan. At the time of death the person's eyes are closed, candles are lit and the covered body laid on the floor. The body should not be left unattended until the arrival of a loved one or the rabbi. The sacred washing of the body should only be undertaken by specific members of the Jewish community. Jewish burials should take place as soon as possible. They are usually held within twenty-four hours of death.

CHRISTIANITY

Christians believe that they will go to heaven when they die. Catholics believe they must repent of their sins in order to enter the full glory of heaven. A priest will pray with the dying and offer Holy Communion, anoint with holy oils and the dying receive the sacrament of penance and reconciliation. It is customary to recite the Lord's Prayer at the time of death.

SHAMANIC WAYS, ANCIENT TRADITIONS

Many traditions, particularly shamanic ones, will welcome the ancestors and invite them to assist with the transition process. They may call in spirit helpers and guides through song asking for help, love and guidance in the sacred passing of that person. At the point of death the space where that person died will be blessed and cleansed through the burning of sage, sacred sound, prayers, and positive intentions.

Space clearing

Space clearing rites will be conducted in many religious practices. These are simple ceremonies to lift the residue of

energies that may have become stuck, making the atmosphere feel heavy in the room where that person has died.
Space clearing is done to clear the energy and to ensure that
the person's spirit has moved on. Sunlight and fresh air will
help remove stagnant energy, so open windows, spritz the
air with essential oils or buy "space clearing sprays" from
any holistic shop. In eastern traditions it is usual to place
a bowl of salt in the middle of a cleansed room, or small
bowls of salt in each corner of the room where energy gets
trapped and can be absorbed in the salt. In Tibetan traditions,
'Tingshas, ancient cymbals, are played to cleanse and uplift
the environment.

To cleanse the space after someone has died I set my inten-
tion by saying "I call upon Divine Love to bless, purify and
fill this space in honour of the passing of . . . (the name of the
deceased). I then sing my song "By the grace of your grace"
and close by saying, "In perfect love and perfect trust this place
is clear of any residual negative energy and is now a place of
peace and love".

"Following the light of the sun we left the old world"

Christopher Columbus

Allowing for your grief

"To weep is to make less the depth of grief."

William Shakespeare

Do not underestimate how heartbreaking it can be witnessing the passing of an elder, someone of whom you may have
grown very fond, thought of as your own family almost,
and now they are gone, and you will be caring for many
others who will be passing over. Acknowledge your grief,

do not become hardened by it, recognise that it is human nature to mourn the loss of the people one has cared for. Do not forget to care for yourself, so **please refer to the self-care chapter** for supportive ideas and exercises to help you. Treat yourself gently, talk to a trusted person, write down your feelings, pursue art or creative projects. Debrief with your colleagues and support each other as you grieve the loss of the elder.

"Never apologise for showing feelings. Remember that when you do, you apologise for the truth."

Benjamin Disraeli

Commemorating and honouring

I feel passionately about how we honour someone after death in a care setting. Ideally they should have felt part of "the family" of the home, but in their death how do you show that they mattered. There have been too many instances where residents who have died in care homes are taken "out the back door" so as to not disturb the other residents; no fuss, no fanfare, erased. In all my trainings I advocate the possibility of carers and nursing staff creating a walk of honour as the body is taken respectfully through the front door. Staff and residents can acknowledge, pay respects and grieve together, giving that elder a heartfelt and respectful send off from their "last home". I know many funeral directors who experience this are very touched.

"Puts your faith back in human nature, it has always felt wrong to be taking out an anonymous body rather than a person that mattered."

George, funeral director

Many carers are unable to attend a funeral service but there are many other ways of commemorating someone's life you might like to try.

- With other carers, or on your own, you could light a candle and dedicate it to the memory of that elder as your own ritual.
- Have a picture of that elder with their favourite flowers next to it and a book for people to write their favourite memories of that elder.
- Have a tea party in memory of the elder, or serve their favourite food at the next meal, play their favourite music, or sing their favourite song together.
- Plant a pot in memory of the older person.
- Create a memorial path with the first names of those that have passed written on stones to line it.
- Create a quilt with each square dedicated to an elder who has passed.
- Hold a memorial tribute for those that have passed.
- Create a mural with their first names.
- Create a tree with hanging pictures of the elders.

"When one of our residents dies, the mortuary men come, and as we're wheeling the body out through the garden, heading for the gate, we pause. Anyone who wants to – fellow residents, family, nurses, volunteers – shares a story or a song or silence, as we sprinkle the body with flower petals. It takes a few minutes; it's a sweet, simple parting image to usher in grief with warmth and care."

Sam, care home manager

CONSIDER

Someone may come into your care home and you know nothing about them and they die overnight, but the one thing you can guarantee is that they will have been loved by at least one person in their life and they will have loved at least one other person too, and that in itself is worth honouring and commemorating.

Thank you

Thank you for all that you have done and will do, the ripples of your compassionate care I believe will be felt in many, many ways. Please understand how you played an important part in each person's final transition. You can reflect on the journey you took with them by asking yourself these questions.

- Did I actively help them to achieve the death they hoped for?
- Did I help them to express their wishes?
- Did I act with respect and dignity?

Recognising that we learn through experience, ask yourself in each situation what you might have done differently. Make a note of any thoughts and ideas to benefit the next person who will be fortunate enough to receive your loving care at the end of their life.

"Each human should die with the sight of a loving face."

Mother Theresa.

APPENDIX

Care planning and documentation

With thanks to contributor Cathe Gaskell, Director – The Results Company

It is a Nursing Midwifery Council requirement to have a documented plan of care. Without a specific document delineating the plan of care, important issues are likely to be neglected and the resident's wishes and choices can be overlooked. Care planning is an essential part of healthcare, but is often misunderstood or regarded as a waste of time. However it is the best way to ensure residents get the care they need whoever may be looking after them.

The care plan has long been associated with nursing and nurses or health care assistants who plan care and write it and keep it updated. It can however be a good idea to involve a range of staff in creating a personalised care plan about your resident. This should include the views of other members of the team as well as the resident and their families where possible. The care plan will include information about the resident, and it often includes a life history or information about past life choices and interests, the resident's profession, hobbies and family as well as their medical information and history. It is important that the care plan reflects not just the current care needs (physical health needs) of the resident but also considers their psychological, emotional and spiritual needs as well.

Care planning could be considered as providing a "road map" of sorts, to guide all who are involved with a patient/resident's care. It is important that the care plans you develop are easy to read for those who deliver them as this will promote consistency when you may not be on duty. In creating a care plan for residents requiring nursing care, the plans you make will mainly relate to difficulties in the Activities of Daily Living (ADL); eating, dressing, toileting, bathing, grooming, transferring, and the care plan will detail how safely the resident can manage these tasks.

You will also need to complete tools that help you to prioritise individual care needs and identify if specific help is needed in areas which could deteriorate rapidly and impact on the health of your resident. Two of the most common tools you could find within the documentation that you need to complete are as follows:

MUST – malnutrition universal screening tool that is used to determine if the resident is malnourished or at risk of malnutrition or obese.

Waterlow or Braden scales – measures skin integrity or how fragile and vulnerable the skin is and the likelihood of pressure ulcers.

It is important to attend training before using the tools and to familiarize yourself in scoring and recording the resident's results accurately.

DoLS

Other important information that may be in your resident's notes is information about The Mental Capacity Act, which allows restraint and restrictions to be used but only if they are in a person's best interests. Extra safeguards, the Deprivation of Liberty Safeguards (sometimes referred to as DoLS), are needed if the restrictions and restraint used will deprive a person of their liberty. These DoLS apply to any resident who lacks capacity to consent to the arrangements made for their care or treatment in either a hospital or a care home (registered under the Care Standards Act 2000) or for whom a deprivation of liberty may be necessary in their best interests to protect them from harm. The assessments need to be completed by a qualified professional and recorded in the resident's notes.

Do

- Keep your documentation up to date, as your resident's health or needs change. Make sure you record these changes in their notes.
- Take time to check the resident's choice in areas of personal care and food. How did they like to dress, how did they wear their hair? What was their favourite recipe? Make your resident's time in the home full of choice and let them make decisions about their care and by whom or how it is delivered.
- Take time to read the notes when you have been off work or you have not worked with the resident for some time. What has changed about them, what do you notice is different?
- Ask for support and training on completing care plans and using the tools.

Don't

- write notes about things you haven't seen or witnessed yourself;
- change or amend notes after an incident has occurred, but make a separate note and sign and date it;
- forget to speak to your resident's family members and friends about their life before they required full time care, so that you understand the person behind the illness or frailty you may see now.

Tips for carers

- Include a recent photograph, as well as past photographs, in each resident's files. It helps identify your residents, it helps staff personalise the care they are delivering and remind them of who the person was before they needed care.
- Make your signature always easy to read as you sign each entry, as the notes are a legal document.
- Always write in black pen and don't use Tippex but cross out instead and sign if you amend the documentation.

Checklist

- Make sure your documentation is personalised and up to date and reflects your resident's current health needs, don't let the information about your resident become out of date.
- File old health information, the information you don't need every day, at the back of the file or have it archived.
- Make sure all signatures are easy to read and dated.

AFTERWORD

Honouring the elders

When I take my end of life workshops I ask carers to think about all those elders in their lineage, their ancestry, that are responsible for bringing them into this world. I suggest that even if they did not have a good relationship with their parents or grandparents, they did give life to them and they in return are giving care and love to others, and that in itself is worth recognising and honouring.

I will often conduct a tree planting ceremony where we plant new seeds in honour, love and gratitude to old lives, those who have gone before, the elders of our elders, our ancestors. After we have planted our seeds in the ground I will share my prayer . . .

As we stand on this sacred land
At this sacred time
May we honour our Ancestors
Those that have gone before,
so that we can be born
into this dear world once more

May we give thanks to
Blessed Mother Earth
Who holds us so tenderly
and shares her beauty
So generously.

We honour and give thanks
to the Standing Ones,
the oaks, the trees
who witness our ceremony
They hold and transmute
Divine Love
and remind us to root ourselves
in love and with love.

We give thanks
to the Winged Ones,
the birds that sing the love
of joy's remembrance,
reminding us
to give voice
to love

We give thanks
to the Waters of the Earth
that lead us back to our rebirth,
and the renewal
of Sacred Ways.

We give thanks
to the bright Golden Sun
reminding us
we are all One

*and to bask
in the warmth
of Love*

*We give thanks
to the gentle breeze
rustling the leaves
on the trees,
reminding us to
let love
be free.*

*And we honour
the seeds
within this holy ground
in this forest where
we have found
a place of grace and peace
where Love Divine
will never cease.*

Thank you for reading *The Carer's Bible.*

May your life in this dear world and the next be filled with opportunities to give and receive love.

BIBLIOGRAPHY

and recommended reading and resources

Bonner, Chris, *Reducing Stress-related Behaviours in People with Dementia*, London: Jessica Kingsley, 2005

Blunt, Leslie, *Music Therapy*, Routledge, 1994

Casledine, G, 'The Use of Language in Nursing Care', *British Journal of Nursing*, May 2008

Department of Health, *The Dignity Challenge*, 2006

Feil, Naomi, *The Validation Breakthrough*, third edition, 2015

Fenwick, Peter and Elizabeth, *The Art of Dying*, Continuum, 2010

Foote, C, and Stanner, C, *Integrating Care for Older People*, London: Jessica Kingsley, 2005

Help the Aged, *My Home Life*, Help the Aged, 2006

James, Oliver, *Contented Dementia*, Vermillion, 2009

Janki Foundation, *Values in Healthcare*, Janki Foundation, 2004

Kubler-Ross, Elizabeth, *On Death and Dying*, Routledge, 1970

May, H, and Perrin, T, *Wellbeing in Dementia*, Churchill Livingstone, 2000

Moon-Willems, Chris, *Relative Matters*, Bookshaker, 2012

Moorjani, Anita, *Dying to Be Me*, Hay House, 2011

Myss, Caroline, *Anatomy of the Spirit*, Bantam Books, 1997

Network Training, *Provision of Activities for Older People in Care Settings*, tribal

Nolan *et al*, 'Quality in Ageing Policy Practice Research', Brighton: *Pavillion Journals*, 2006

Parnia, Sam, *What Happens When We Die*, Hay Publishing, 2007

Pool, J, *The Pool Activity Level (PAL) Instrument*, London: Jessica Kingsley, 2008

The Royal College of Nursing, *Spirituality in Nursing Care*, 2010

Sheard, David, *Enabling*, The Alzheimer's Society, 2007

Smith, P, *The Emotional Labour of Nursing: How nurses care*, Basingstoke: Palsgrave McMillan, 1992

Sogyal Rinpoche, *The Tibetan Book of Living and Dying*, Rider, 1992

Speyer, Josephine, and Wienrich, Stephanie, *The Natural Death Handbook*, Random Books, 2003

Waring, Amanda, *The Heart of Care*, Souvenir Press, 2012

Warner, Felicity, *Gentle Dying*, London: Hay House, 2008

Warner, Felicity, *The Soul Midwives' Handbook*, Hay House, 2013

Woods, Robert T, *Alzheimer's Disease*, Human Horizon Series, 1989

Spirituality and Ageing, London: Jessica Kingsley, 1998

FURTHER READING

Helpful websites, links and organisations

Action on Elder Abuse
Works to protect and prevent the abuse of vulnerable older people
www.elderabuse.org.uk
Free helpline 08088088141

Age UK
Information, support and grants for all aspects of elder care and support for those looking after someone with dementia, information about all aspects of end of life planning and care as well as what to do when someone dies
www.ageuk.org.uk
Advice line 08001 696 565

Alternative Therapies in Health and Medicine. 6 (Nov 1999): 49-57.
Music therapy increases serum melatonin levels in patients with Alzheimer's disease.
Http://www.alternative-therapies.com/index.cfm/fuseaction/archives.main

Alzheimer's Association
Late stage caregiving
Http://www.alz.org/care/alzheimers-late-end-stag
e-caregiving.asp

Alzheimer's Association
Music, art and Alzheimer's
Http://www.alz.org/care/alzheimers-dementia-music-ar
t-therapy.asp#music

Alzheimer's Foundation of America
Education and care: music
Http://www.alzfdn.org/educationandcare/musictherapy.
html

Alzheimer's Society Canada
For family members and caregivers: suggestions for the late
stage
Http://www.alzheimer.ca/en/Living-with-dementia/
Caring-for-someone/Late-stage-and-end-of-life/For-famil
y-members-and-caregivers

Bright Copper Kettles
Activities for older adults
www.brightcopperkettles.co.uk

Carers UK
a comprehensive range of information for carers on their
website
www.carersuk.org
Free carers line 0808808777

Celebrant
amandawaringevents.com

Celebrants
www.UKCelebrants.org.uk

Crossroads Care
Britain's leading provider of support for carers and the people they care for
www.crossroadscare.org.uk
Tel 0845450 0350

Death Cafés
At death cafés people get together in a relaxed setting to safely and informally discuss death along with tea and cake
www.deathcafe.com

Depression Alliance
Helps people suffering from depression, it offers information and advice as well as a network of support groups
www.depressionalliance.org
Tel 08451232320

Dignity in Care
For support and online forum
dignityincare.org.uk

Dying Matters
Information on what to expect during end of life care and ideas for funerals and support
www.dyingmatters.org

Elderly Parents
Provides information for adult children caring for elderly parents
elderlyparents.org.uk

Final Fling
An informative website looking at death and dying
www.finalfling.com

Hospice Information Service
www.hospiceinformation.info

Hospice of the Heart
For information on supporting the dying in a holistic way
www.hospiceoftheheart.com

Macmillan Cancer Line
Information on cancer and Macmillan nurses
www.macmillan.org.uk
Tel 0808 808 0000

Marie Curie Cancer Care
Information on cancer care and Marie Curie nurses
www.mariecurie.org.uk
Tel 0800716 146

National Association for Mental Health (MIND)
Offers support to people in mental distress and their
families
www.mind.org.uk
Free advice line 02085192122

The National Association of Complementary Therapists in Hospice and Palliative Care
www.nacthpc.org.uk

The Natural Death Centre
Provides information about woodland burials, cardboard
coffins, living wills, funeral wishes forms and do it yourself
funerals
www.naturaldeath.org.uk
Tel 01962712690

Princess Royal Trust for Carers
A comprehensive site providing information advice and
support services to carers
www.carers.org
Tel 08448004361

Revitalise

Offers special Alzheimer's holidays for people with dementia
and their carers, which are subsidised by the Alzheimer's
Society
www.revitalise.org.uk
Tel 08453451970

Sane

A mental health charity, which supports those with anxiety
or depression
Tel 08457678000

The Transitus Network

A network of people involved in supporting those that are
dying in a sacred way
www.transitus.co.uk

Women's Royal Voluntary Service

Find out where your nearest local one is, they offer a choice
of services, including visiting schemes, home delivered
meals, volunteer drivers etc.
www.wrvs.org.uk

FILMS AND PRODUCTS BY AMANDA WARING

What Do You See?
This powerful award-winning short film has been acknowledged as one of the most valuable tools to highlight dignified and compassionate care for the elderly. It is used around the world for inductions into caring careers. The film follows a day in the life of an elderly stroke victim, Elsie, played by Virginia McKenna, who makes a silent, but heartfelt, plea to her carers to "Look closer . . . see . . . me".

Home
Starring Virginia McKenna, Home looks at Elsie's arrival in her new care home as she struggles with the transition and mild dementia. This poignant six-minute film helps us understand the emotional journey of an older person during this time.

No Regrets
A daughter visiting her elderly mother in hospital leads to startling revelations about caring, grieving and dying. This sensitive film helps you support and understand the relative's perspective and reminds you that it is never too late to tell someone you love them.

The Big Adventure
Using interviews, poetry and humour, this uplifting and inspiring film examines end of life care and our attitudes towards death to stimulate debate and provide a varied selection of concepts and beliefs. This film is used in many hospices and care settings to challenge and transform care and to embrace the spiritual needs of those who are dying.

The What Do You See? training pack.
The pack consists of a work book with a DVD of Amanda's films supporting the exercises and a CD Rom containing the handouts required. This motivational pack provides 50 hours' worth of training around dignity.

I am near you CD
This beautiful CD of Amanda's songs and meditations is used in care settings as a comforting presence to those who are maybe dying alone or when care staff and family are unable to be present. Amanda's soothing melodies and healing words help to calm, to uplift and to alleviate a feeling of being alone.

Amanda's award-winning films on dignity and end of life care are available from the online shop on her website www.amandawaring.com

ALSO BY AMANDA WARING

Available in ebook and as a paperback edition

THE HEART OF CARE:
DIGNITY IN ACTION:
A guide to person-centred compassionate elder care

The Heart of Care is a life-changing guide for carers and caring professionals, asking them to question their attitudes and behaviour and to re-connect with their compassionate natures to help those in their care to lead rich lives. It provides a guide to valuing elderly people and those who care for them, involving the older person in decision making, providing a positive social environment, enriching the lives of those being cared for while leaving staff feeling more valued in their work.

"Ways that could transform how we deliver care . . . promote better elder and end-of-life care."

'The Lady'

Including the creative use of role-play exercises, anecdote and practical advice to uplift, motivate and educate carers, this is an essential guide to developing the skills and awareness that NHS staff and carers need to support an ageing population. **The Heart of Care** embraces principles that will change our society into one that truly cares for, and nurtures, elderly people with dignity.

"A practical, supportive little book that would be of use to anyone caring for older people . . . its common-sense approach is refreshing."

'Nursing Standard'

The Heart of Care is a rallying cry to improve the physical, emotional and spiritual care of the elderly; a timely, vital and inspirational message for our times.